2/26/14

Judy — THANK $

Mary Yoo
keep Lov doing
well & helping
so many

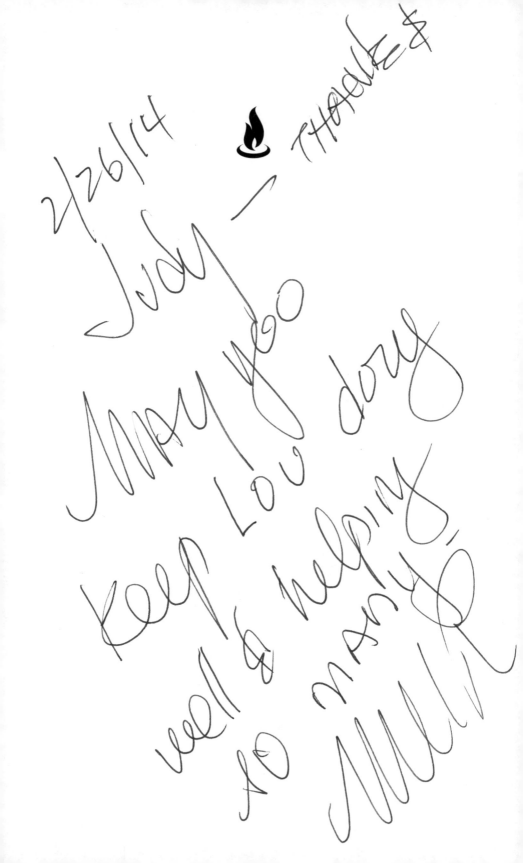

Also by Michael F. Roizen, M.D.

RealAge: Are You as Young as You Can Be?

*The RealAge Diet: Make Yourself Younger with
What You Eat* (with John La Puma)

*Cooking the RealAge Way: Turn Back Your Biological Clock with
More Than 80 Delicious and Easy Recipes* (with John La Puma)

*The RealAge Makeover: Take Years off Your
Looks and Add Them to Your Life*

*The RealAge Workout: Maximum Health,
Minimum Work* (with Tracy Hafen)

The *YOU* Series, Cowritten with Mehmet Oz, M.D.

*YOU: The Owner's Manual: An Insider's Guide to the
Body That Will Make You Healthier and Younger*

*YOU: The Smart Patient: The Insider's
Handbook to Getting the Best Treatment*

YOU: On a Diet: The Owner's Manual for Waist Management

*YOU: Staying Young: The Owner's Manual
for Extending Your Warranty*

YOU: Being Beautiful: The Owner's Manual to Inner and Outer Beauty

*YOU: Having a Baby: The Owner's Manual
to a Happy and Healthy Pregnancy*

*YOU: Raising Your Child: The Owner's Manual
from First Breath to First Grade*

*YOU: Losing Weight: The Owner's Manual
to Simple and Healthy Weight Loss*

*YOU: The Owner's Manual for Teens: A Guide
to a Healthy Body and Happy Life*

*YOU: Stress Less: The Owner's Manual for
Regaining Balance in Your Life*

*YOU(r) Teen: Losing Weight: The Owner's Manual to
Simple and Healthy Weight Management at Any Age*

THIS
IS YOUR
DO-OVER

The 7 Secrets
to Losing Weight, Living Longer,
and Getting a Second Chance
at the Life You Want

MICHAEL F. ROIZEN, M.D.
with TED SPIKER

SCRIBNER

New York   London   Toronto   Sydney   New Delhi

Scribner
An Imprint of Simon & Schuster, Inc.
1230 Avenue of the Americas
New York, NY 10020

First Scribner hardcover edition February 2015

SCRIBNER and design are registered trademarks of The Gale Group, Inc.
used under license by Simon & Schuster, Inc., the publisher of this work.

For information about special discounts for bulk purchases,
please contact Simon & Schuster Special Sales at
1-866-506-1949 or business@simonandschuster.com.

The Simon & Schuster Speakers Bureau can bring authors to your live event.
For more information or to book an event, contact the Simon & Schuster Speakers
Bureau at 1-866-248-3049 or visit our website at www.simonspeakers.com.

Manufactured in the United States of America

1   3   5   7   9   10   8   6   4   2

Library of Congress Cataloging-in-Publication Data

Roizen, Michael F.
This is your do-over : the 7 secrets to losing weight, living longer,
and getting a second chance at the life you want / Michael F. Roizen, M.D. ;
with Ted Spiker ; foreword by Mehmet Oz.
       pages   cm
       Includes index.
   1. Self-care, Health.   2. Health.   3. Vitality.
   4. Weight loss.   5. Rejuvenation.   I. Spiker, Ted.
   II. Oz, Mehmet, 1960– writer of foreword.   III. Title.
       RA776.95.R65   2015
   613—dc23   2014049798

ISBN 978-1-5011-0333-9
ISBN 978-1-5011-0335-3 (ebook)

To those who have taught so much with their Do-Overs;
to my family, who have allowed me the time to learn;
and to those who want a Do-Over so they can serve more

Contents

Foreword

We all know that many things can heal your wounds: medication, surgery, time. Modern medicine now has the power to fix so many health problems with what seems like a flip of the switch. This dose, that procedure, this shot, that bionic body part—you got it, we can cure it. While everyone certainly knows that we can't cure everything, it's absolutely true that we live in a time of unprecedented medical breakthroughs that have the power to improve and extend lives.

We've gotten pretty good at the fixing.

But you know what? That's no way to live. Get a problem, fix a problem. Have a wound, stitch it up. Feel an ache, pop a pill. In fact, there's something dramatically wrong with the problem-solution approach to the way that we, as individuals, treat our health. By relying on the medical advances and experts to band-aid our problems, we've relinquished our power—our power to live strong, healthy, energetic, and satisfying lives.

While I've spent most of my career in fix-it mode ("heal with steel" is what we surgeons like to say), I've made a fairly dramatic change in where I put my medical energies these days. Much of that is thanks to Michael Roizen. I have flipped my own switch, spending my time talking to people about shifting the medical equation—going from a problem-solution paradigm to a prevent-the-problem way of thinking. Why? Because that's where the real power is: creating a healthy body to prevent health issues from developing in the first place, and having the strength and resiliency to fight back when they do come up.

That's what Mike has spent so much of his career doing: studying data, working with patients, redefining what it means to be young and healthy. I, of course, knew Mike from his days of working on RealAge, the phenomenon that taught America that we were only as old as our bodies acted, not as old as the calendar said. But after we were introduced by a mutual friend, Craig Wynett, who had a vision for our partnership, Mike and I decided to collaborate on the *YOU: The Owner's Manual* series of books—a series that taught folks about anatomy and biology, as well as what steps they could take to improve theirs. Through our relationship, I have learned that there is nobody—*nobody*—more passionate about helping others get well and get healthy than Dr. Michael Roizen. He walks the walk (quite literally ten thousand steps a day) and talks the talk as the Chief Wellness Officer of the Cleveland Clinic and "the Enforcer" on *The Dr. Oz Show*.

And that's one of the many reasons why I'm so excited about this book, *This Is Your Do-Over*. Mike has taken his main message—changing your life through changing your behaviors—to assure you that no matter what mistakes you've made in the past, you can get your body back. And I don't mean that in the bikini-by-tomorrow kind of way. I mean it in the biological live-a-long-life kind of way (though the exterior benefits will come, too, if you follow his steps).

By explaining the biology about how you have the power to control the way your genes work, Mike takes you through scientifically proven tactics to help erase your health mistakes (and maybe counteract some of your genetics) to get the body and life that you want. The best part of *This Is Your Do-Over* is that the plan Mike outlines is manageable: every action can be worked into your life, no matter your personality, your genes, your preferences, your lifestyle, anything. These seven Do-Over deeds, as he calls them, essentially work as the pillar strategies that will get you where you want to go. I've seen it work on the show for people who just needed a little help, and watched Mike help those who were in great need of a second chance.

In this book, you'll find insights from the medical data, as well as anecdotal evidence from Mike's patients and his own life. Together they will serve as your ammunition to fight any of your health challenges.

Above all, I hope what you take from this book is that it's not too late. It's not too late to find solutions. It's not too late to make changes. It's not too late to live the way you want to. It's not too late to find the passion and purpose in your life—and allow them to be the drivers of good health choices.

It's not too late.

Best of all? Your body already knows that.

All you have to do is help it find its way.

Mehmet C. Oz, M.D.
New York-Presbyterian/Columbia University
Medical Center heart surgeon and Emmy
Award–winning host of *The Dr. Oz Show*

INTRODUCTION

Change of Direction

In just about every aspect of our lives, we accept—no, we embrace—the notion of second chances. Our children learn from the mistakes they make. Our bosses don't fire employees for every screw-up (unless perhaps it involves NSFW photos on the official company Twitter account). Movie directors say "Take two." Golfers get mulligans. Artists throw away canvases that don't have the right shades of blue. Politicians, celebrities, and athletes bounce back from embarrassing public faux pas. Husbands, wives, partners, and friends work their way out of the doghouse. Shoe-eating puppies can do the same. For the most part, we accept that life is imperfectly beautiful—and that part of the way we grow, develop, and learn is through trials and errors, and more trials and more errors. We accept that life works like that in all areas except one: our health.

When we make mistakes in *this* domain, we beat ourselves up. When we're not living the way we want, we crawl into a hole and set up camp for the long haul. We don't forgive ourselves. And when we find ourselves living a life that we don't want to live, we medicate ourselves with sugary treats the size of the Roman Colosseum.

And then for good measure we scarf down another colossal indulgence, in despair over the first.

We have to stop treating our health mistakes as an all-or-nothing, once-and-for-all sentence. We have to think of our health the same way that we think about most other aspects of life.

We have to stop thinking that we must live forever with the choices we once made or with the genetics we think that we're stuck with. We have to stop this mentality that once we've slid down the slippery slope of cheese fondue, there's no ladder to get us back up.

You have to embrace the fact that you *do* get a second chance. We—you—can reverse health problems associated with inactivity, overeating, addictions, depression, much of your genetics, and most anything else. You can live life with high energy and happiness no matter the nature of your health concern. No matter how long you've had it. No matter what kind of shape you're in. No matter what you've tried in the past.

You can have a Do-Over. You deserve a Do-Over.

This—right now—is your Do-Over.

The payoff: by learning to incorporate seven simple principles into your life, you can erase virtually all of the damage that your body may have sustained. And by doing that, you live not only longer but also better—with a stronger body, a sharper mind, a more fulfilling sex life, and so much energy that Congress might even consider you a fueling strategy for a seven-state area.

As the Chief Wellness Officer of the Cleveland Clinic and someone who has dedicated his career to helping people make 180-degree turns with their health, I know that many of you feel desperate for that total transformation. Just look at today's health statistics; many people are in deep, deep trouble. More than two-thirds of American adults are overweight or obese. Nearly one-third of Americans will have diabetes by the year 2050 if current trends continue. About 600,000 die of heart disease every year, consisting of nearly a quarter of all deaths. There are a predicted 1.7 million new cases of cancer that will be reported in 2015. And the scariest part is perhaps this: even if you're not one of those statistics, you could well be on your way. We're a society that eats too much, moves too little, stresses all the time, and doesn't get enough sleep. And like a cyclist pedaling against traffic, we're headed in the wrong direction.

I choose not to get depressed by those numbers. I choose to go right to you—to metaphorically high-five you, fist pump you, hug you—and tell you that it's not too late.

No matter what kind of lifestyle you have led, no matter what bad habits you may have, no matter if you're a smoker or a sugar snorter, you have the ability to get on track, start over, and reboot your body so that you can live a healthy life. You can change the way your genes function through your lifestyle choices. You do not have to be destined to certain health outcomes because your parents were on the same path or because you think you've already done irreversible damage. So forgive yourself. Move on; you can have a Do-

Over. The science shows that you can change your body from the inside out.

In my job (not just at the Cleveland Clinic but also as "the Enforcer" on *The Dr. Oz Show*, author of the *RealAge* series, and coauthor of the *YOU: The Owner's Manual* series), I have seen it time and time again. People can and do turn around their health, and that turns around their enjoyment of life.

In this book, I'm going to teach you how to do your Do-Over. It's your second chance—your decision to change your health destiny, so that you live your life with energy and happiness, and not as one of the statistics I mentioned a few moments ago.

My career has been about helping others find wellness in their lives. In this book, I boil down all that I have learned about the most important areas of wellness and teach you the seven simple secrets to a better life. These are the tools to help you start over, whether you have one bad habit to change or need an entire life overhaul. I will address nutrition, exercise, sex, stress, sleep, the brain, and all of the other areas that contribute to total-body wellness. Using the most cutting-edge data, anecdotes about people I've worked with, and the advice that has worked for the thousands that I have personally coached, I will give you the formula for a simple yet effective Do-Over to reclaim your health—and your life.

When I was nine years old, I was the sickest I could ever remember: horrible sore throat, feverish, sick to my stomach. I felt like my body had been buried in the back of a garbage truck and obliterated into a crumble of mush. Soon after

I came down with the symptoms, the family doctor gave me a shot (which I now presume was penicillin) to treat a severe case of strep throat. Within hours, I felt better. I felt good. I felt like myself. I know that I was only nine, and I know that kids change their minds a zillion and a half times about what they want to do with their lives, but I can tell you very clearly that this was the moment I knew I wanted to be a doctor. My nine-year-old self said, "If I could help people feel better and make sick people healthy *and* get paid for it, wow, that's what I want to do!" And I've never strayed from that goal: to help people get healthy. That's what I love doing (which, by the way, is also one of the secrets to your Do-Over: finding and cultivating your own passion in life).

I started my medical career in anesthesia and critical care, and by looking at data about how we could improve our patients' health outcomes, I learned a valuable lesson: we could dramatically reduce the rates of mortality and other adverse effects of surgery if we could care for younger people. That is, if we could somehow rejuvenate our older patients' bodies, their outcomes would be more favorable. The evidence is indisputable: the younger a person's body, the better it can handle the stressors presented to it. Well, that would seem on the surface to be nonsensical data, useful perhaps for aliens or folks with time machines—there was obviously no way in the world to turn a sixty-five-year-old into a fifty-five-year-old.

Or was there?

Indeed there was. My mission was figuring out not how to make people live longer, but how to make them live younger—so that anyone could have the body (biologically speaking) of someone five, ten, fifteen years younger than his or her calendar age. That was the basis for my work in RealAge and virtually every other wellness project I've worked on—not about extending your life in the classic way of thinking about it (Let's live to ninety-five!) but about extending the quality of your life (Let's live until ninety-five, while feeling like we're a fraction of whatever age we actually are!). Through this goal, I learned where the data are, and I learned what makes our bodies break down, and what heals them. Essentially, I wanted to invent a biological time machine that could take your body back to a place that real life could never bring you. I wanted to make you younger.

And that's what the Do-Over is about: helping you lose weight, stop smoking, have wonderful relationships, and jump into life rather than hide from it.

So how will we get there? I've broken this book into seven essential Do-Over deeds that will help you get your body back. Within each of those deeds, you'll find the seven most essential things you need to know about that particular area. (There is something magnificent about the number seven, right?) Within each chapter, I'll take you through a mixture of information, strategies, inspirational stories, and hard data to give you all the essentials for taking control of your body and your health. I'll also mix in a little behind-the-scenes information about my own life so that you can better understand how these strategies can work into yours.

The literary bookends of those seven chapters come in the form of two sections that will serve as the foundation and action for the rest of the book. For starters, I'm going to take you through a mini medical school: a quick look at some of the biological processes that you should have a handle on before we begin. Don't worry, you don't have to memorize the difference between the ilium (the pelvic bone) and the ileum (the final segment of the small intestines), and there will be no test to take at the end. I wrote this section so that you really get a visceral understanding of how the body works, because when you do that, you can better understand how those things will change your body for better or worse. I don't like to throw around words like *inflammation* and *epigenetics* and *carbohydrates* without giving you a primer on what they are and how they work. This basic knowledge will fully prep you to make the most of your Do-Over.

In the final section of the book, I'm going to give you my ultimate Do-Over preparation plan. It's easy to implement and will get you headed in the right direction within just seven days. (I sense a theme!) We'll use those seven days to fully prepare you to embrace the actions you need to take to get your Do-Over going.

Finally, I want you to remember this fact: of the research we have, it appears that very few people practice five of the healthiest behaviors for achieving and sustaining wellness. These are: (1) walk thirty minutes a day, (2) eat healthy, (3) don't smoke, (4) have a waist less than half your height, and (5) drink alcohol only in moderation. Case in point: only 3 percent of US nurses—the heart of our health force—engage in all five behaviors. Yet if you practice them regularly, you will lower your risk of having a major adverse health event—heart attack, stroke, cancer—by 80 to 90 percent compared with those who don't.

Those statistics tell me one thing: we have a long way to go, yet we have much to gain if we can get there.

I hope that this is what my book helps you do, and that my seven secrets to achieving your Do-Over are all the direction you need. I'll mix information with inspiration, science with stories, and motivation with a must-do action plan that will help you turn your life in the direction that you want.

And while you may be reading this alone, thinking about all of your challenges alone, and assuming that you have to go at it alone, know this: when it comes to your Do-Over, *alone* is a dirtier word than even Louie CK could come up with.

In fact, my very first Do-Over deed is all about teaching you to change your mind-set—including thinking that you have a solo journey ahead. I'll be there with you for part of it, but your second mission will be making sure to bring someone along the way. Your first mission?

Enroll yourself for a few minutes in my mini medical school, where I'll teach you about how your body works, so that you can learn how to make it work even better. The payoff—a smaller size, longer life, sharper mind, and better sex—is waiting for you.

So let's go!

THIS
IS YOUR
DO-OVER

Mini Medical School

Your Biological Cheat Sheet

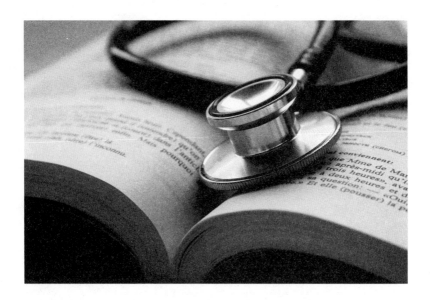

When students are in medical school, they assume quite a few roles. They're part language scholar, learning a vocabulary that only they can speak and understand. They're part walking encyclopedia, as they learn about every body part, medication, and disease. They're part detective, as they learn how to piece together symptoms and figure out what might be wrong—from the common problem to the rare one. And, of course, they are part healer and part teacher, as they learn not only to fix problems but also to prevent them. At a cost of seven years (including the barest of residencies) and upwards of $250,000 to become a doctor (after college), it's a big investment.

For you—someone who needs to know a bit about your body to maximize your chances of a successful Do-Over—it'll cost much less. Now by no means am I implying that after reading the next few pages, you'll be equipped to scrub up and perform a lung transplant or a self-colonoscopy. But in this chapter—your mini medical school—I want you to learn the basics of how your body works, especially when it comes to the key areas involved in your Do-Over. Why? Because I firmly believe that for you to truly "get" that these choices are great for you, you have to understand why they matter at a visceral level—yes, the blood and guts of it. If you can "get" how a certain action works to give your body that Do-Over, you're more likely to do the things that help and avoid the things that hurt. And once your body starts to rev better, you're more likely to keep these new habits, especially if you know how and why they make a difference.

The following curriculum is short and fast, but it's also very important. We'll cover the big-picture issues, conditions, and concepts that lay the biological foundation for your Do-Over.

So take a spin through, learn the basics, and get ready to enjoy your Do-Over. And remember, in this course, there's no test, no reason to cheat—because the only person you'd be pulling a fast one on is yourself.

Genetics 101

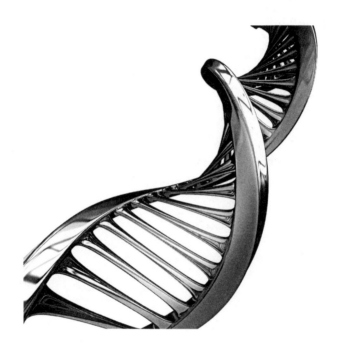

You may already know your genes have a lot to do with aspects of your personality, what you look like, and why you may be more prone to store excess lasagna on your thighs or your arms. There's no doubt that genes are the key ingredient in the concoction that your mother and father created; they make you, well, *you*. But it would be a mistake to blame your health on your genes. Genes lay the foundation for who you are, but they don't *dictate* who you are. The data show that only one-quarter of your health comes from your genetics, while three-quarters comes from your lifestyle. That's essentially what this whole book is about: giving yourself license to have your Do-Over, no matter what genetic hand you've been dealt.

Because physicians put so much emphasis on factors such as family history, most people assume that means there's nothing they can do about the fate of their health. Normally, when we think about genetic traits, we think about qualities that can't be changed or are essentially predetermined, such as height or eye color. But when you take certain actions—smoking, eating well or eating poorly, exercising, managing stress or not—you actually manipulate your genes to manifest themselves in certain ways, thus controlling and influencing the biological processes in which they're involved. Yes, you have the ability to manipulate your genes. Doing that means you can turn them "off or on" in the way they function. That's the foundation for a field called epigenetics—that is, your ability to influence how your genes express themselves.

Your genes act as protein factories or controllers for those factories. Turning on a gene means that you make more of the protein than that gene normally makes. (All genes really do is help make proteins or monitor or modify the actions of other genes.) Turning off that gene means that protein and its effects are diminished or absent from your body. And yes, your choices do just that: turn your genes on or off. In addition, you greatly influence the function of the proteins they make through your actions. For example, a protein called hemoglobin, found in red blood cells, travels the circulatory system, transporting oxygen to your body's tissues. Well, having too much simple sugar (found in white carbs, baked goods, etc.) in your diet brings about high blood sugar levels, and that, in turn, causes sugar to attach to your hemoglobin proteins, preventing them from releasing oxygen normally. *That* produces such outcomes as nerve pain. So poor food choices lead to a change in how your body operates, which can lead to ill health or the feeling of numbness or even big-time pain.

The Hand You've Been Dealt

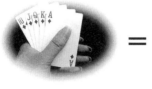 =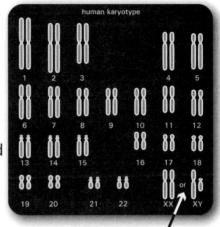

human karyotype

All of your genetic information is found in 23 pairs of chromosomes, which are made of DNA. Almost every cell of your body has this *exact same* set of DNA.

What about this 23rd set? XX = female, XY = male.

What Genetics Determine

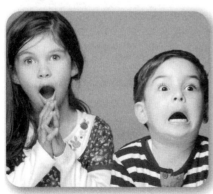

Genetics determine factors such as eye color, height, facial features, and predisposition to certain diseases. (They may also be one small ingredient of many that influence personality.)

What Genetics Don't Determine:

Your Health Destiny!

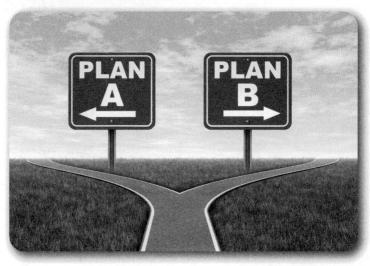

Change the Function of Your Genes

Epigenetic studies
reveal that
you can turn
your genes
off or on.

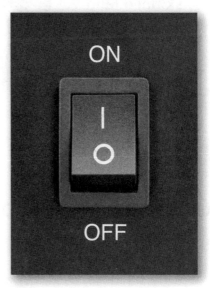

Change the Function of Your Genes

Two ways:
- Your choices change your genes to be either read (and produce a protein) or skipped (and the protein that gene would direct isn't made).

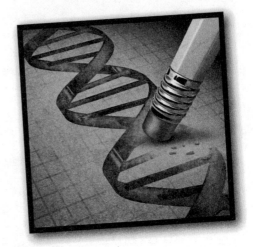

Change the Function of Your Genes

- You can keep your telomeres (tiny parts at the end of DNA strands) long. Long telomeres mean you can keep repairing your body.

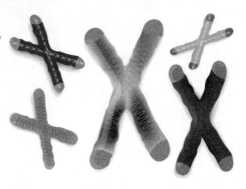

The Way to Think About Epigenetics

Your body forecasts its future based on what you're telling it. Your genes adapt to those instructions.

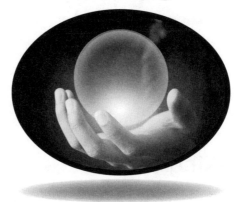

The Lifestyle Effect

You can steer your body to be more efficient and less prone to wear and tear with choices that repair and heal your body, not break it down.

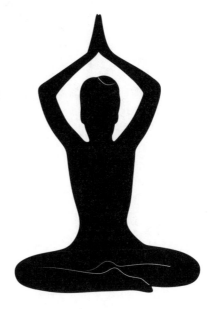

Passing It On

Even better,
the changes
you make can
positively
impact your
offspring and
generations
to come.

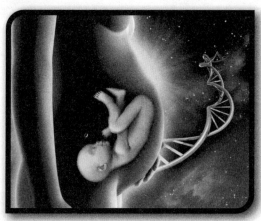

Inflammation 101

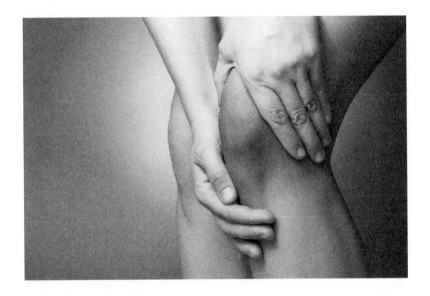

This word gets tossed around like pizza dough: "Causes in-flammation." "Careful of inflammation." "Uh-oh, I think he has inflammation." But what does that really mean?

Inflammation, by definition, isn't a bad thing. In fact, it can be a really good thing. When your body is injured, inflammation is part of the immune response—that is, your body's healing mechanisms, such as signaling your white blood cells to rush to the injured area to help repair it. Similarly, it's what happens when you skin your knee; your immune response scouts out the problem, then signals your body to go fix it and close the wound to prevent nasty gunk from entering your body. When you get an infection, bacteria or viruses provoke inflammation, which beckons one type of your immune cells. Those immune cells I.D. the invader and then call forth your killer immune cells to come to that spot and attack those nasty bacteria and viruses. When they're all done destroying the bad guys, your immune cells commit suicide so that they don't keep attacking your own cells or organs in what is referred to as an "auto-immune process."

This is how we want your body to act. The problem starts when acute inflammation, the temporary type, turns to chronic inflammation. One way chronic inflammation occurs is when your immune response doesn't shut off as it's supposed to; the cells don't commit suicide. So all of those chemicals and cells keep on fighting, after the fight should be over. That's when you get further swelling, pain, joint issues, compromised organs and systems, and many processes that cause or contribute to other diseases and conditions, including autoimmune diseases. You may not see or even "feel" this kind of internal, chronic inflammation per se (though it can manifest through pain and conditions like arthritis). But make no mistake: chronic inflammation isn't something to ignore.

So what causes chronic inflammation? All kinds of things, such as certain foods, smoking, stress, and obesity. Fat in your belly doesn't just sit there and store calories—it produces proteins that cause, and increase already present, inflammation. Even just eating more than 4 ounces of red meat a week or one egg yolk a week changes the bacteria inside your intestine to produce a molecule that promotes inflammation and thereby ages your arteries, the tubes that carry oxygen-rich blood and nutrients to every cell and organ in your body. That could mean heart attacks, memory loss, strokes, kidney disease, impotence, and wrinkles down the road (see cardiovascular issues, below). And that inflammation promotes arthritis and cancer. On the other hand, there are plenty of things that reduce inflammation; you'll learn more about them throughout this book.

What Is Inflammation?

Your body sends in immune cells to attack any-thing that it perceives as a threat.

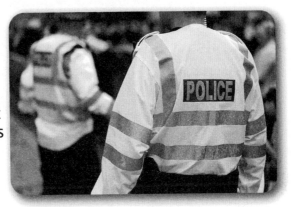

Is That Good?

Yes, for short periods of time, such as when your body is healing from an infection.

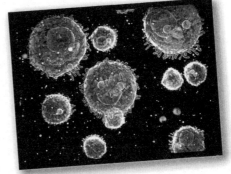

Your immune cells
- kill the invaders and
- start to repair damage.

So What's the Problem?

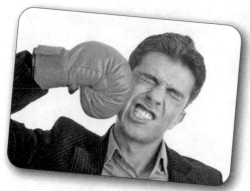

If your immune response goes on and on and on, your immune cells can start attacking your own healthy tissues.

What Does It Affect?

Inflammation can damage your:
- joints,
- heart,
- circulatory system,
- kidneys, and
- brain.

It can also trigger cancer cells.

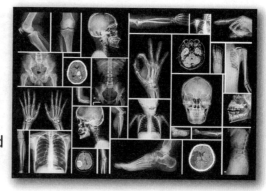

How?

If your body attacks itself when there's nothing to attack, it's like friendly fire in your body.

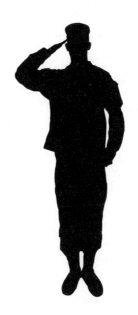

Do You Feel Inflammation?

You can, through flu-like symptoms, general pain, swelling, and fatigue or loss of energy and exhaustion.

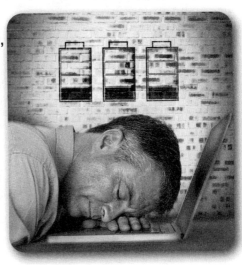

Inflammation Can Be

All that swelling and immune activity—that puts pressure on your body's systems, causing them to break down.

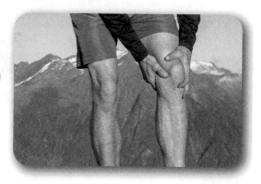

Keeping It in Check

Healthy habits don't give your body a reason to want to fight.

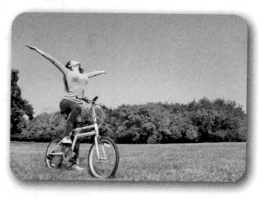

Cardiovascular Issues 101

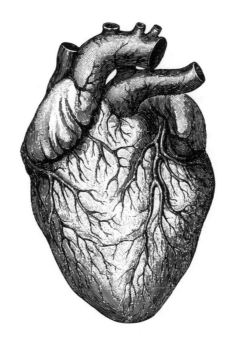

You already know that docs spend years studying the intricacies of the heart in medical school. And considering that the heart isn't just the subject of pop songs and rom-com movies, I know that devoting only a few words to how your heart works seems like I'm glossing over your body's blood pumper. But for our purposes, there's just one concept I want you to master: it's all about blood flow. Every one of your body's organs, tissues, and systems needs blood delivered to it—that's how everything functions, because blood carries oxygen as well as the body's primary energy source: sugar. No blood, no function. No function, no good.

Many things, of course, need to be working properly to guarantee adequate blood delivery to your tissues. That includes your heart, as it pumps blood throughout your whole body. For now, though, I want to concentrate on your blood vessels—the tubes through which your blood travels. That's where much of the damage and danger lies. Here's how: when something (smoking, bad foods, and so on) damages the inner lining of your arterial walls, it creates a sort of nick in the blood vessels. That nick, as you can imagine, damages the vessel, because its integrity is compromised. Even more potentially damaging is what happens next: your body sends in lousy low-density-lipoprotein (LDL) cholesterol to try to patch up that nick—sort of like spackling over a nail hole in the wall. As that plaster builds and builds, and becomes inflamed, it turns into plaque and clogs up the blood vessel—to the point where either blood slows or can't get through. That's what contributes to high blood pressure: your heart has to pump harder to get blood through your blood vessels to your tissues. So you develop higher blood pressure as your body tries to force blood around and past blockages. Chronically elevated blood pressure is called hypertension.

As you can imagine, those blockages are the root of all kinds of cardiovascular-related problems. If blood can't get to your brain efficiently, you'll have memory issues or even a stroke. If blood can't get to your private parts, you'll have sexual-function issues. This process is linked to your previous mini med course topic, inflammation. Chronic inflammation in your blood vessel walls leads to larger nicks and plaques and hinders function of the endothelial cells that line your arteries; both further restrict your circulation. And that means more and more problems getting adequate blood flow. If blood can't get to and from your blood vessels nourishing your heart, you'll risk having a heart attack. This is why we doctors are so concerned with your blood pressure numbers and inflammation inside your arteries. We want—we need—for blood to move freely throughout your body, not just to get the BP number down, but because it influences just about everything else that happens in your body. So getting your Do-Over really means doing what you can to reduce the damage to your blood vessels in order to enable your entire cardiovascular system to work at its highest level possible. And the great news about your Do-Over is that, if you are like most, you can even reverse what's happened before.

Blood Vessels: Your Transportation System

Arteries + veins
+ capillaries =
60,000 miles.
That's 20 times
across the
United States.

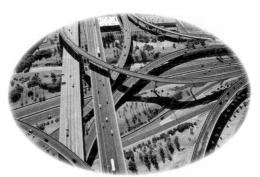

Heart: Your Transportation System's Engine

Your heart
pumps 2,000
gallons of
blood every
day—700,000
gallons every
year.

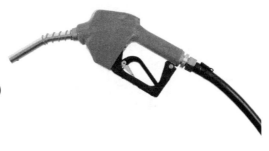

Blood Delivers Nutrients/Fuel to Body

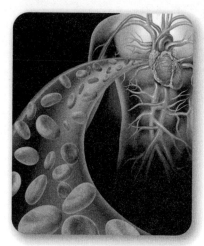

Blood delivers glucose and oxygen to power your organs and tissues.

Blood Delivers Nutrients/Fuel to Your Body

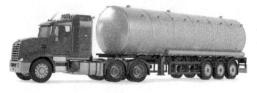

This delivery system is the reason why you can think, move, have sex.

For Circulation to Deliver Fuel to Power Your Cells, Vessels Need to Stay Clear

When there are obstructions, it is harder for blood to get through. That causes high blood pressure, or worse.

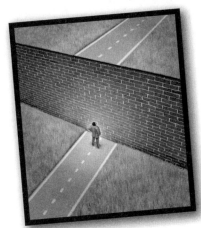

For Your Body to Work, Vessels Need to Stay Clear

Even worse: blockages mean nutrients—even oxygen—are slowed or stopped, leading to:

- heart attacks,
- strokes,
- memory loss,
- erectile dysfunction

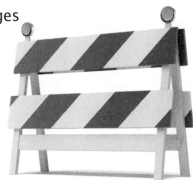

Clean Living = Clean Vessels

Healthy choices prevent or even reverse vessel-damaging blockages.

(Taking on a buddy, the right exercises and foods, stress management, and all of the other deeds you'll learn throughout the book!)

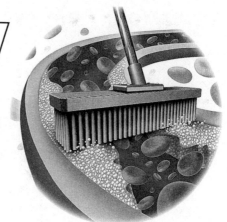

Great Living = Clean Vessels

Blood pressure = a most important number and indicator of your overall vessel health.

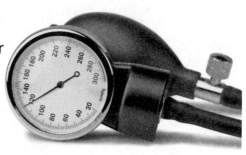

Ideal:
- 115/75 under age 60.
- 125/85 if you've had high BP and are over age 60.

Fat Storage 101

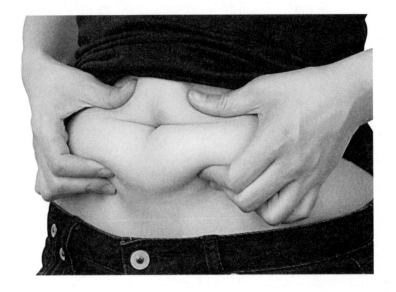

You can boil down the whole biological process of fat down to one word. No, not *cheese*; it's *energy*. Your body needs energy to function. Every organ and every process needs some kind of gasoline or electrical cord to power it. Unlike the world, where there are all kinds of energy sources (wind, solar, nuclear, oil), your body gets its energy from one place: food. If you have no food, then you have no energy source. And with no energy source, your tissues break down quickly. Eventually all of your organs and systems will shut down, and you'll die. Food provides that energy in the form of a calorie. Every calorie provides nutrients that your body uses to help its systems and organs work. Remember from our previous lesson that the energy is shuttled through your body to all of those places via your blood. Your body burns that energy through outward processes such as movement, and also through all of the internal and "invisible" processes, like thinking, digestion, and other organ functions. All of these jobs require calories. (In fact, your brain is actually your biggest energy user, if you are typical.) So in an ideal world, your body would burn the exact amount of calories that it needs to create a sort of equilibrium—use what you need every day, burn what you use, and then repeat for your entire life. But biology (and environment) can't be that precise. There's not a perfect way to easily regulate the inflow and outflow of calories. And in today's society, with our abundance of food and far fewer of us doing physical work (at least when compared to a hundred years ago), we consume far more than we burn.

Your body, harkening back to the days when most of humanity lived in perpetual famine, decided long ago that rather than expel all of the excess calories via bodily waste, it would store some in the form of fat, in case you needed energy in times when no food was available.

Unfortunately, our bodies don't know there's food at every corner nowadays, so they keep that fat anyway—and keep it and keep it and keep it—unless we can find a way to burn it off. The reason why that's so bad is not only because belly fat is toxic to our adjacent organs, but also because fat triggers so many of the unhealthy processes we just talked about: it damages arteries, causing high blood pressure, high lousy LDL cholesterol, and harmful inflammation, and promotes type 2 diabetes as well as many forms of cancer.

Calories In and In and In

When you eat, your body takes in calories in the form of proteins, carbo-hydrates, and fats.

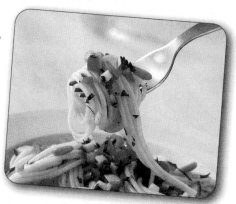

How Do We Get Fat?

Your body takes those nutrients, converts all excess into glucose, and uses it to power all of your body's functions.

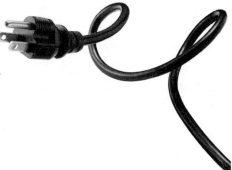

How Do We Get Fat?

When you take in nutrients that aren't used for fuel or for building tissue right now (or that aren't discarded through poop, and so on), your body stores them as fat—an evolutionary mechanism designed to make sure you survive in case you run out of food later on.

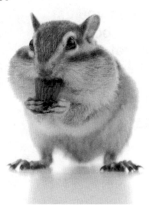

How Do We Get Fat?

In other words, when you eat an excess of nutrients, you store that excess as fat.

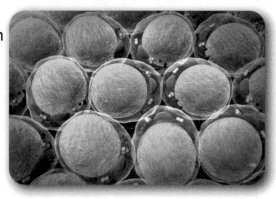

Your Fat Cells

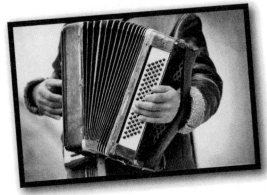

You rarely change the number of fat cells you have. You mostly make your current fat cells grow or shrink.

Belly Fat Is the Worst Fat

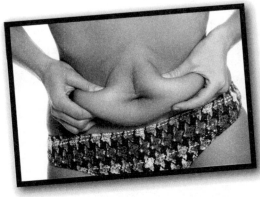

Fat that is stored in your belly is toxic to organs for two reasons:

1. Location: it pumps bad compounds into neighboring organs (thigh fat, not so much).

Belly Fat Is the Worst Fat

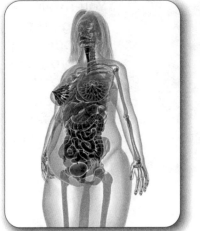

2. Fat in your belly pumps compounds that cause inflammation in the rest of your body.

Issues of Obesity

Eating certain fats as an energy source is fine. *Storing* too much fat by eating in excess—whether fat, sugar, or protein—messes with the chemical processes in you.

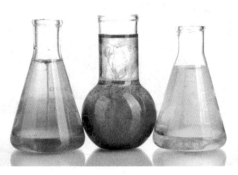

Diseases Related to Belly Fat and Obesity

That extra fat messes up hormonal processes, increases resistance to insulin that contributes to diabetes, and promotes inflammation leading to blood flow issues, arterial aging, arthritis, and cancer.

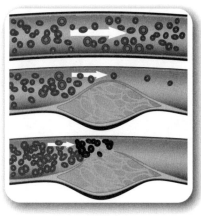

Burn Baby Burn

You can get rid of fat by eating less so you don't continue to add to your stores, and by burning it off through moving more.

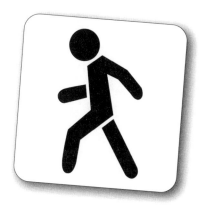

Diabetes 101

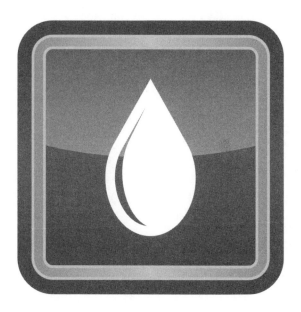

If I were writing a book like this maybe thirty or forty years ago, I might not even discuss diabetes, let alone highlight it as one of the key biological issues that you need to know about. We used to consider diabetes largely a juvenile disease (that's called type 1 diabetes), but with obesity rates skyrocketing, we have to talk about type 2 diabetes (the adult-onset kind, but even kids get it now). Type 2 is the one that's associated with overeating and can lead to all kinds of heart and vascular problems and other health conditions (so much so that we might term this section Obesity 101). Here's how it works:

You remember from your fat-storage lesson how your body needs fuel and how that fuel is shuttled throughout your body? Well, that fuel comes in the form of a sugar known as glucose. It's not only sugar in the way we think of it in terms of table sugar or dietary sugar; all foods—proteins, carbohydrates, and fats—get converted to glucose to be used for energy. Typically, your pancreas secretes a hormone called insulin into your bloodstream. That insulin acts as FedEx and delivers glucose from your bloodstream into the inside of cells throughout your body's muscles, tissues, and organs. When you overeat, that raises the amount of glucose in your blood—and it needs somewhere to go. Your body does the equivalent of adding more delivery trucks by secreting more insulin, but at some point, you just overburden the deliverer, and the packages have to go somewhere else. This is called insulin resistance. All of that excess floating glucose attaches to other substances, in a process called glycosylation. This weakens the junctions between the cells that line your arteries, so the inner walls of your arteries develop nicks. As that happens, you repair those nicks with the fatty streak of unhealthy LDL cholesterol. But it's not normal for your body to have that LDL cholesterol there, so your defense system sends in inflammatory cells to attack that fatty streak, causing more inflammation, raising your blood pressure, and doing all kinds of bad stuff.

You can see where the tipping point is: you have to control your circulating blood sugar by not overeating to maintain an insulin-glucose balance and prevent damage from extra glucose. Worse, consuming too much aspartame, sucralose, acesulfame, and saccharin—the zero-calorie sweeteners that we know as Equal, Splenda, Sweet One, and Sweet'N Low, respectively, and which also sweeten our diet foods and sodas—seems to change the bacteria inside your intestine to produce proteins that add to insulin resistance. These inflammatory proteins further increase blood sugar, further weakening the junction between the cells lining your arteries, increasing nicks, increasing fatty streaks, increasing inflammation in your arterial walls, and making the problem worse. So how do you deal with this? The answer is in chapter 3.

The Hormonal Process

Your pancreas secretes
insulin to take glucose
from your blood into
your cells to power
your body.

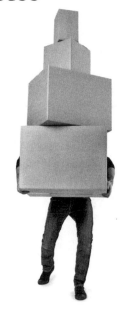

Hormonal Disruption

When you flood
your body with too
much food from an
addiction (or just
because), that over-
loads your body.
Your hormones try
to keep up. Initially
you secrete more
insulin to try to
overcome insulin
resistance.

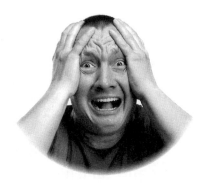

Insulin Resistance

Eventually the insulin you secrete is made less effective at taking glucose from your blood and delivering it into your cells. This is the result of belly fat and the inflammation it causes.

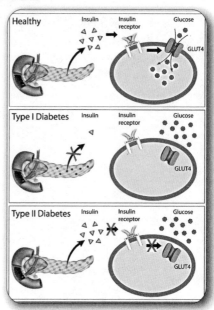

Diabetes

All that unaccounted-for glucose circulates in your blood, making your proteins less effective, causing damage to blood vessels and damage to many other tissues.

Brain Function 101

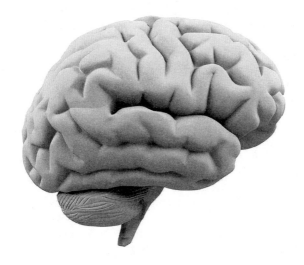

As is the case with almost any of our mini med school topics, you could spend years studying the subject. That's no different when it comes to the brain—perhaps the most majestic and mystifying organ you have. It controls how you think, remember, love, feel, act, and everything else you do. (It's your number one sex organ, too.) So there's a lot to cover, and there's a lot to think about when we talk about preventing aging of your brain.

Certainly the biggest concern most people have revolves around memory—making sure that you keep your sharpness, your cognitive function, and your ability to remember everything you need to function. The way you build and maintain that kind of memory power is through chemical and electrical connections in your brain. Your brain is filled with neurotransmitters: little buggers that relay information from one brain cell (neuron) to another. The more you use those neurotransmitters, the stronger the connection between the nerve cells that send the messages and the other nerve cells that receive them. As you build these connections, your brain gets more powerful. It's how you learn things and get good at those things. It's how you remember things. (The more you read it, the more you know it.) The more you move from one area to another, the better your mental GPS. (Heck, in 2014 they even awarded a Nobel Prize to the scientists who figured out that your brain really does have its own internal spatial memory and tracking system.) On the flip side, if you don't use those connections, they get weaker and weaker—until you eventually lose them. This is why I preach the "Use it or lose it" mantra: you really do need to continue to build those connections to keep your brain functioning at optimum health.

The Learning Pattern

To learn information, your body creates and cultivates connections between neurons, especially in your hippocampus.

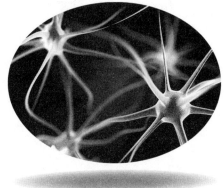

Use It or Lose It

To keep the connections strong, you have to reinforce them with repeated use.

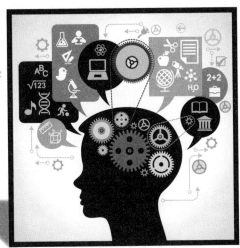

Rx: Challenging Your Brain

It's why one of the best exercises you can do is to constantly attempt to learn new tasks.

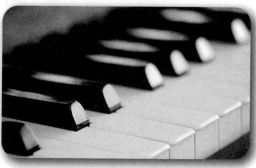

Use That Brain Muscle...

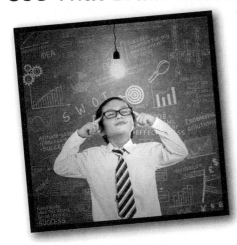

That's why memory is like muscle: the more you work at the connections in your brain, the stronger they are.

...And Use That Muscle for Your Brain

The more you exercise your body, the happier your brain will be. Exercise releases feel-good hormones, and high-intensity exercise actually encourages brain growth.

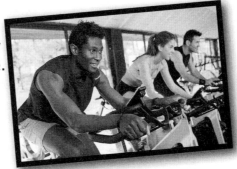

Stress Response 101

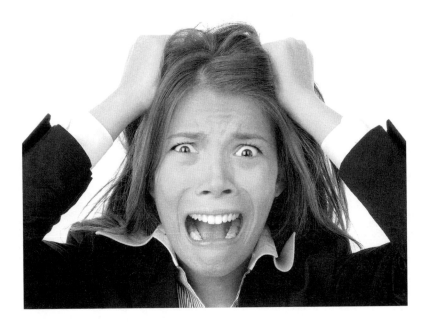

Most of us think two things when it comes to stress: one, it's bad; and two, it's more of a feeling than an actual biological process. Wrong on both accounts. The fact is that stress is actually designed to help you; back in the days of the woolly mammoth, the elevated heart rate and blood sugar levels caused by your response to a stressful event rushed blood and energy to our muscles so we could escape attacking tribes or tigers. That stress was helpful to get us to fight or take flight. It was also fleeting. Once the threat was gone, so were the high blood sugar and elevated heart rates. But now that we're in times when the occasional tiger in the wild has been replaced by the ever-present tigers in the office/family/carpool lane, that means that your stress levels may actually never wane—and those chronically elevated blood sugar levels and heart rates chip away at your health. So some stress isn't bad; it's just that a lot of sustained stress is. Here's how it works biologically: when you're faced with a stressor, your brain (specifically your hypothalamus, the section of your brain that produces these hormones) releases corticotropin-releasing hormone (CRH), which then stimulates your pituitary gland to release adrenocorticotropic hormone (ACTH) into your bloodstream. That hormone is what signals the adrenal gland atop each kidney to release the stress hormone cortisol, which then facilitates the release of epinephrine (also known as adrenaline) to give you the juju to defeat the stressor. I know, I know: that's a heck of a lot of stimulation. This whole cascade of events is called the stress circuit, and it lies at a place called the hypothalamic-pituitary-adrenal (HPA) axis. When adrenaline and cortisol levels are elevated, they age your arteries, destroy connections in your hippocampus (the brain's memory coordinating center), and damage your immune system—hurting not just your happiness levels but also the insides of your body.

Hormonal Processes

When your body has a stress response, hormones such as cortisol and adrenaline are increased as your power boosters.

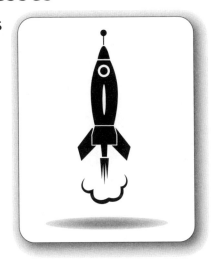

Fight or Flight

Those hormone responses are from the days when stress was a woolly mammoth attacking. Your body wants to save you. So it raises your heart rate and blood sugar, and increases blood flow to muscles to give you the best shot at surviving that attack.

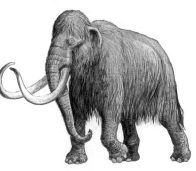

Where It Turns to Trouble

In chronic responses of high stress, your body can't handle it. That results in blood vessel damage, increased glucose, decreased immune responses, and other results of hormonal disruption.

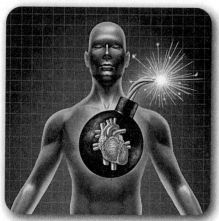

Engage in Relaxation Response to Help You Manage Your Response to a Stressor

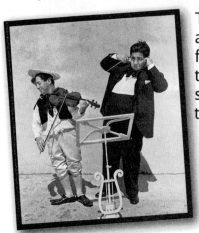

To quiet the hormonal and chemical battle-field, you must manage the source(s) of the stress or your response to the stress(es).

Pain 101

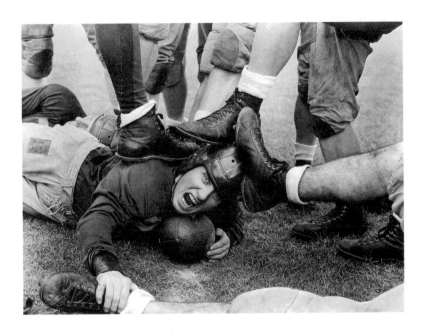

Pain is to the body as pornography is to the Supreme Court: it's hard to define, but you know it when you see it (or feel it, in this case). That's because there are a million types of pain—whether from an acute situation, like stubbing your toe, or from a chronic situation, such as experiencing weeks and weeks of lower back pain. Like stress, pain is also a bit misunderstood—because pain is actually a good thing (which sounds blasphemous to say to someone who experiences a lot of pain). It's good because pain acts as the signal to communicate to your control board, "Houston, there's a problem," and you need to do something about it—like your body's smoke detector or the oil light in your car. If your security system can warn you of a problem before there's a disaster, then that's better than the alternative. Pain is that warning system.

How do you feel pain? Your body senses pain through two sets of nerve endings in the skin that transmit pain. Fast ones have a thick, fatty sheath of myelin around them, which speeds the transmission of pain sensations to your spinal cord and your brain so that you can react faster when the brain tells you to get out of there pronto. Slow nerve endings, without that myelin jacket, produce burning or deep pain.

Almost every tissue has this system to alert you to take care of the problem. As you know, there are various levels of pain tolerance—that is, two people can be exposed to the same exact stimuli and sense the pain differently. That's because several factors influence how we feel pain. Some are biological (gender, age, genetics), some are psychological (how we cope individually with a stimulus), and some are even social variables (such as how different cultures respond to pain).

All of this makes pain a very difficult area to study, but we do know that some chronic pain is caused by or made much worse by some of our lifestyle choices. Factors like tobacco, inactivity, food choices, and untreated stress are all associated with heightened chronic pain.

Pain Is Damage Felt in Tissues and in the Brain

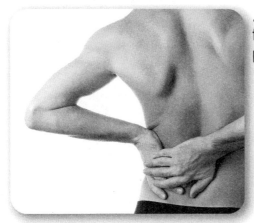

...But it varies from person to person.

Pain Tolerance

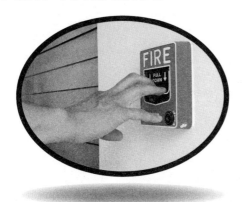

Sometimes pain tolerance isn't a good thing because it shuts off your natural alarm system.

Your Degree

Congratulations! You've earned your mini medical degree. While there will be no residencies, board exams, or actual treatment of patients, you now have the basic knowledge to really get to know how your insides work—and how the things that you do every day can change your systems for better or worse. While I can't offer you a white coat and stethoscope, I do hope you apply your newfound knowledge to your life (and help teach others while you're at it). Now that you've taken the first step on your Do-Over journey, there's only one thing left to do: go for it.

You can have a Do-Over. Forgive yourself. Forget about your past. Take care of the present, and you'll take care of your future.

Friends with Benefits

7 Things You Need to Know
About Nature's Best Medicine

Today's health care landscape is full of amazing developments that can heal your wounds, fix your problems, and make you healthier with tools crazier than we once could have imagined: robotic arms to perform surgery; chips that categorize your genes; phones that can take your pulse or record how well you slept; pills that lower your lousy cholesterol, quiet your aches, and improve your sex life. We live in a time when the possibilities for efficiently and effectively preventing and treating health problems are as endless as an infinity pool. I have little doubt that decades from now, people will look at this era as one that revolutionized health and medicine. The hope that we can develop the cure-it-all tools that will help us live better, healthier, and longer is a very real one. As someone who has dedicated his life to helping people have fun, live healthfully, and reverse the damage they've done throughout their lives, I am excited about the potential of these emerging technologies to improve the dreadful health statistics we see every day.

But you know what? Right now, you have the power to improve your health and prevent disease with a tool that's free and doesn't require any new technology at all: a buddy. That buddy can come in the form of a spouse, a friend, a family member, a virtual friend, a coach you pay, anyone. (In this book, I'll use the word *buddy* interchangeably to mean that one special person.) Whatever form this person takes, the point is that having a buddy involved directly in your wellness goals will make you substantially healthier.

It sounds simple, but for many people it isn't. That's because so many people approach their health issues with a sense that they should keep everything to themselves, bottling up their questions, their fears, their achievements, and sharing with no one. If they only knew that having a buddy they can count on is a major influence on their overall health, they'd figure out problems that no medicine can even begin to solve. This is especially true for the set of people who already are dealing with health issues or are on their way to having some major health problems. These folks need that buddy in their Do-Over because many times they feel as if there's nothing they can do themselves, that there's no way out, that they're all alone, or that they don't want to burden others with their problems. So their health problems get worse and worse, when, in fact, if they just used the power of a buddy, they could kick-start the Do-Over process and get headed in the right direction.

Through both the anecdotal evidence I've seen year after year, and the hard data that are abundant in the medical literature, it's absolutely clear that this is the game changer. Recruiting a buddy is the most important choice you can make to heal your body and reverse damage you may have done. It sounds simple. It even sounds improbable. Yes, it was a surprise to me. How in the world could one special person be more powerful than decades of medical research or the expertise of our finest doctors? The buddy system works by helping you make good choices, by coaxing you to be smart about your behavior, and by cheering or jeering you when you do the tangible things that have an influence on the way your body works. This may feel like a hug-everyone platitude, but I assure you it's not. There's real science that shows the power of relationships can help change the biology of your body, and that you can have fun while doing so. Relationships do this through a number of mechanisms, and they work for a number of reasons, all of which I'll explain in this chapter.

Truth is, buddies are multifunctional: they're your power strip, because they can provide you energy when you need it. They're your security guard, because they can help you stay accountable when you slip off track. They're your light pole, because they illuminate knowledge when you have gaps. They're your safety net, because they're a secure place to tumble when you're struggling. And ultimately, if you choose wisely, they're your dance partner, because they work with you rhythmically and instinctually to move through life with grace, vitality, and a smile.

One of the first times I saw this phenomenon in action was when I wrote *The RealAge Diet* in 2001. As part of the program, we set up an online buddy system that would match people with similar interests, personalities, and goals so that they could have one-on-one relationships to discuss issues and ask each other questions—as well as provide each other support just by being there. About 290,000 people signed up to find a match; six months after their first pairing, 166,000 people were still logging on and staying in contact with their buddy.

That experience showed me three things: One, if that many people needed to reach out to find a buddy, then an even larger number of people were missing this piece of the puzzle. They didn't have that buddy in their lives, and they knew—or felt—that a buddy would help. Two, it showed me how well the buddy system worked. If that many people kept up with the program—and thus developed real relationships—then we knew it would have the power to help people heal physically and mentally. Three, it showed me that all kinds of buddies could do the trick. Your buddy could be someone you meet in person or online. It could be someone you're close to or someone you have never even met. That's a powerful message, especially for people who do not feel they can share their worries with their families, for whatever reason; maybe they don't want to scare their family, or maybe they do not feel they get support from their family. In this chapter, I'll show you some of the science and reasoning behind choosing your buddy, as well as how it helps you with your Do-Over.

As we start, just keep in mind that no matter what your current health condition—whether you're trying to treat a problem or prevent one—the best medicine doesn't neces-sarily come from the drugstore (unless you meet your buddy there). It comes from having one other person in your life who understands your wellness goals and is as committed to helping you achieve them as you are. The potency of this medicine is off the charts, and the side effects are very few.

In fact, it may very well be the only remedy in the world that should be prescribed to everyone—regardless of age, gender, race, size, family history, or condition.

#1 | The Buddy Effect Has Tangible Health Benefits

Natalie is an intensive care nurse in a lung transplant division at the Cleveland Clinic. When she first joined the lung transplant team, she started working with a man who was overweight, on three blood pressure medications, and who needed to get in shape. His kidney function had deteriorated to the point where he was close to needing to go on dialysis; this man who worked at an organ transplant unit was well on the way to making it on the transplant list himself.

Natalie had already gone through the Cleveland Clinic's stress reduction program, and had learned a lot about how to handle daily pressures and manage her body. The clinic encourages all of its employees to wear pedometers, so the two of them would talk about and share their latest walking numbers. They walked more and more, and Natalie's buddy even started going to a local track as he took on a new mission to walk consistently; eventually they agreed to challenge each other. They decided to see if she could run a clinic-sponsored ten-kilometer race faster than he could walk a five-kilometer race. The challenge was all in good fun, and it served as a way for them to push each other, and hold each other accountable for making sure they got in the daily activity they needed. Natalie, who had been a runner in college, beat her coworker's time by a few minutes, but the result of the race didn't matter. What mattered is that the man lost twenty-five pounds—and he said later that he never would have done it without the encouragement and help of his buddy Natalie. "I asked him if someone he didn't know had done the challenge with him, would he have kept it up, and he didn't think so," Natalie said. "It was knowing me and not wanting to let me down—that type of camaraderie." He really got a Do-Over: after he walked with his buddy and lost the twenty-five-plus pounds, his kidney function improved to near normal. A miracle? No, just the Do-Over that happens to many when they become physically active.

This is the kind of Do-Over story I witness time and time again, as I've run various weight-loss, smoking-cessation, and overall wellness programs. The common thread—besides doing the healthy eating, stress management, and activity—was that the successful people all had a buddy in their quest to lose weight, or stop smoking, or lower their blood pressure, or alter whatever it was that annoyed (and threatened) them. The key word in the last sentence is *all*.

You don't have to trust the anecdotal evidence to know that the power of the buddy system is real. This concept was studied by University of Chicago and now Harvard University researcher Nicholas Christakis, who found that social networks have a viral and "contagious" nature; that is, we take on the habits of the people around us. In short: your friend walks, you walk; your friend eats doughnuts, you eat doughnuts.

This may happen, in part, because of something you have in your brain called mirror neurons, which fire in your brain when you observe someone performing an action—these fascinating neurons fire as if you were actually doing the very behavior you observe. Basically, mirror neurons cause us to automatically rehearse the actions of the people around us for our own future use; they could, in part, explain why we take on the same habits of our personal communities.

In essence, it's a very subconscious reaction: what your friends do, you do. But that subconscious effect is not the only way your friends' behavior influences your own. You most certainly use the words and actions of friends to help guide your actions more consciously as well. If you have a buddy who asks to play tennis, you're more likely to do that than watch a movie and gorge on twelve boxes of Junior Mints; your friends have a direct influence on your decision making. That's not even taking into consideration all of the psychological benefits that can happen—the supportive words, the coaching, the kick in the butt—when you actually talk through issues and obstacles. No matter the influence, the evidence is clear that strong relationships can mean having a stronger body.

Some more evidence:

People who feel lonely have a 14 percent higher risk of premature death than those who don't feel lonely. (In comparison, poor people's risk of dying prematurely is 19 percent higher than it is for those not living in poverty.) The researchers looked at the link between "feeling lonely" and health issues that might be relatively easy to identify as influencing premature death. A couple of insights surfaced, including the fact that loneliness can raise blood pressure, lead to less restful sleep (sleep problems are associated with making you look and feel older than your biological age), and increase your body's production of the potentially damaging stress hormone cortisol.

Research shows that marriage is good for your heart, and not just in the Valentine's Day box of chocolates kind of way. One study found that married men experienced healthier blood pressure changes than single men. According to another study, the chance of suffering a heart attack or stroke doubles within the first thirty days after a spouse dies. Some research indicates that this may be caused partially by partners being less likely to take their medications in the month after a spouse's death, but there's also evidence that losing a spouse is associated with harmful changes in blood pressure, heart rate, and other physiological functions.

It's not enough to be married, though. One study using computed axial tomography, better known as a CT scan, showed that those who felt they had a supportive spouse had less calcium buildup in their arterial walls, meaning they were at lower risk of having heart troubles. Couples that were ambivalent about how supportive their spouses were exhibited higher calcium levels in their vessels.

Though many of these studies use married couples as their subjects, the findings extend beyond the bounds of matrimony; good support systems make you healthier. While it's not always clear what mechanism is at work, there's enough data to show that those in supportive relationships have better health outcomes—both because of biological changes when stress is lessened and because of the positive behavioral changes that a partner influences.

#2 | It Can Help Overcome Our Most Destructive Addictions

If we posed the question "What's most destructive to our overall health?" some might say cigarettes. Some might say overeating. Some might say too much stress or too little sleep. Blame this, blame that, blame the fact that some restaurants serve *appetizers* that have two days' worth of calories. But I think if you had to put an umbrella term over all the things you do that cause serious health problems, most of them would fall in the categories of destructive habitual behaviors or all-out addictions. Though the prevalence of cigarette smoking is on the decline, our addiction to sugar and other forms of junk food is at the heart of not only the obesity problem but also the conditions associated with obesity, such as heart disease, many cancers, and type 2 diabetes.

The reason why addiction is so powerful and pervasive is because, well, addiction is one of those forces that we feel we don't have any control over. It's true that, in a lot of ways, when it comes to being addicted to something, the only thing at play is the reptilian part of our brains—the part that makes us just react and act without reason or thought toward the past or the future. See sugar, eat sugar. See cupcake, eat seven of them. Addiction stops us from thinking—and just gets us acting.

How? Addiction is a complex phenomenon, but it all starts when a substance (or behavior) actually creates physical changes in your brain. This physical change is related to the neurotransmitter chemicals that bridge the gap (synapse) between brain cells, enabling messages to be relayed from one brain cell to the next. The physical change also involves creating new pathways or connections, called neuropathways, between brain cells. Those changes in your brain make you feel like you're starving for that substance or behavior and that you'd die without it.

Let me explain how: when you're addicted to something, you begin to crave it because a key neurotransmitter, such as dopamine, has signaled your brain to feel pleasure. You want more, and you develop a habit to get more. You keep up that process of needing more until it becomes an addiction. You repeat the behavior to get that biological IV hit of dopamine. But your body adjusts, so over time you need more and more to achieve the same pleasurable feeling. So you consume more and more of whatever it is that once gave you that feeling—for instance, more and more chocolate chip cookies. And then something bad happens: your body can't make enough dopamine, so you keep reaching for the behavior that you hope kicks it in, but now with less or no effect. In the case of sugar, you reach for more and more, never satisfying the dopamine hit, but packing on extra calories that (1) eventually turn to fat, (2) create exhausting energy highs and lows, and (3) can put you at risk of developing diabetes. You need a buddy to help you get over that reptilian craving for sugar—you need a buddy to help you get your Do-Over. Why?

As you establish and continue new behaviors, you're actually laying down new neural pathways—new tracks, so your brain remembers what it's supposed to do. Essentially, you are programming your brain to do the behavior. Now, yes, it's true that some people are genetically predisposed to addiction—they have what we call addictive personalities. But whether an addiction is genetically or environmentally based, the problem is that you have a hard time overriding that reptilian part of your brain that causes you just to act rather than to think first of the consequences of your actions.

What the heck does this have to do with the buddy system?

Get this: according to the data, our most effective anti-addiction drugs cure the craving only 3 percent to 5 percent of the time. When we add in an element of support through a second party, a buddy, that number soars to 35 percent. Tenfold. Incredible! One of the most powerful brain-related problems we have (addiction) can't (yet) be outsmarted by medication, but it can be by your buddy.

We don't know exactly how, but likely it's due to a combination of factors. For one, there's the benefit of having someone around who understands your addiction, who can talk to you when you're tempted, who can occupy your mind and provide support when you're in tough spots, and who can suggest solutions or alternatives that get your mind above that reptilian reaction. That is, your friend elevates you past "can't think, must act" status, so that you can get to the human response of "think of an alternative." Once you

can overcome that urge, your brain pathways are pruned—
to get a long-term Do-Over. We see this model used in a
number of popular addiction-related programs, such as Al-
coholics Anonymous (AA) for alcohol addiction and Weight
Watchers and similar diet programs that utilize the power of
social networks.

The buddy system may also work because a social network helps you to release chemicals in your brain that
counteract your brain's impulse to seek out dopamine fixes
through unhealthy behaviors. When you feel a close bond
with someone, your neurons release into your bloodstream
the powerful feel-good chemical oxytocin, which makes
you feel intimacy and community; it's the same hormone
that bonded you to your mother when you were born.
When you're in good relationships, romantic and otherwise,
you release oxytocin, and that is part of what helps you feel
good.

When you think about what addiction is all about, chemically speaking, it's a race to feel good. Because your brain
has been taught the behavior that will make you feel good,
that's the action that you reach for. But it certainly seems
that with an increase in meaningful relationships, you can
sort of whip up on that process and give your brain another
kind of high—a high that can get you to turn destructive
behaviors into productive ones. The result: you become
addicted to the positive feedback, the relationship, and the
progress that you make because of it. Your buddy helps you
get that Do-Over you want and deserve.

#3 | Pick Your Perfect Partner

Carol started her weight-loss journey in September 2011. Her husband had tried to lose weight many times—losing 20 to 30 pounds, but then quickly gaining it back. He topped out at 293 pounds and had kidney stones once a month, on average. At one point, he was put on a restricted diet of just 1,200 calories a day, and yet he gained 3 pounds in two weeks. (Good lesson there: don't restrict calories too much, or else you'll teach your body to want to store fat because it senses you're not getting enough!) Once he met with a nutritionist (his buddy at that point) and changed his eating habits, he started losing weight—and he ended up losing more than 100 pounds in seven months. Carol, "not wanting to get behind," joined in and lost 80 pounds herself—dropping from 216 pounds to 136. Even better, their teenage daughter lost more than 50 pounds too.

Now, Carol and her family had one another, and their buddy system worked well. In the end, they ate better and felt better. "We learned how to rid our bodies of the foods that were keeping us down and overweight," she said. "I never in my wildest dreams thought I would be able to lose that amount of weight and feel as good as I do." They forgave themselves and one another for past failures, and they didn't feel any shame—nor should they have. Those failed attempts were just failed attempts, and had nothing to do with their ability to succeed now. As for her husband, he hasn't had a

kidney stone in a year, and he can walk miles without breaking a sweat, whereas before, he would break a sweat merely
walking from the car to the store. A family Do-Over!

As is the case with any successful Do-Over story, many
factors played a role. They ate better, they exercised, they
managed stress, and they learned the behaviors that would
help them lose the weight. But here's the point: look at how
many times the husband failed. It wasn't until the whole family got involved—three people with similar goals, supporting
one another in their quest—did it work for the long term.
They succeeded in a total family Do-Over because they had
one another as buddies. And I imagine for many of you,
your immediate partner or family member may work out
really well. It's convenient, you already love and support each
other; you don't have to build a relationship while changing
your body. That's great. But it's not a requirement to have
your spouse, partner, or family member be your buddy.

In fact, there are lots of reasons why it may *not* work.
Sometimes partners are at different health stages, and it can
be hard for both sides to really relate if one is super fit and
healthy and one is not. There's a danger of the buddy system
turning into the I'm-superior-to-you system (or, likewise,
the I'm-inferior-to-you system), which isn't good health-
wise or relationship-wise.

For example, Val and Calvin met in the armed services,
when both of them were fit. But with each of her two
pregnancies, Val gained weight and could never get back to
baseline, going from 135 to 185, to 165 to 215, then down
again to 185. When I saw her fifteen years after the first
215, Val had gone back up to an all-time high of 224, she

had early type 2 diabetes, and she was frustrated. She hadn't forgiven herself—she was ashamed and felt she'd been defeated by lousy cookies and ice cream—and she was afraid that her weight was destroying her marriage. Calvin, you see, had stayed fit and had tried to be her buddy, but it hadn't worked. We started Val with the various programs that you will learn in this book, so that she could change her lifestyle and get that Do-Over. She understood that the past was the past; she forgave herself, as she saw that her self-worth did not have to be tied to her past habits. She started on our daily email exchange—where she found her buddy, me. One of the indicators for whether participants in our buddy email program are going to be successful with their Do-Overs is if they email daily. (This daily email needs to happen to help you follow your plan—helping you increase your number of steps from week to week, without trying to get you to do too much, too soon, which can lead to injury, frustration, and eventually giving up. This is where most failure happens—because people are discouraged. It's much better to take progressive steps.) Val started and has continued perfectly. Her buddy nudged her and helped her overcome obstacles. She lost 14 pounds and 3 inches from her waist in the first month, and after two months, she'd reduced her diabetic medication and lost 18 pounds. My bet is that she'll get to her desired 155-pound goal, get rid of her type 2 diabetes, and sustain her Do-Over and her relationship with Calvin.

Of course, it's a sad reality that not everyone is in the best of relationships. You may not get the right support from your partner if other aspects of your relationship aren't clicking.

The bottom line is that you have to choose a buddy who's going to work for you, who will be there over the long term (so you can sustain your Do-Over), who wants to serve as your buddy (both giving and receiving support), and who is worthy of your trust. Your buddy can be a family member, a friend, a coworker, a coach, a trainer, or a neighbor. It can even be someone you met online, or someone who lives across the world with whom you communicate electronically. Even a paid coach can work wonders, as long as he or she has the knowledge to help you and is willing to be your buddy and care about you and your success. The possibilities are endless, but that doesn't mean selecting your buddy is an easy decision. I've seen many "buddies" (well-meaning or not) sabotage the health of their "friends." True friends don't let friends age prematurely. They keep each other younger. Ultimately, you want someone who is willing to take the time to listen—even if it's just by responding to your email or text crying, "Help! The cheese cubes are staring me down!"

So how do you choose? Often, you'll just know that one person who's always been there for you, and it may be a matter of making a call or sending an email or text, asking if he or she will help you along the ride to health. Ideally, I believe the best buddies have these four qualities:

1 They listen to your story to understand the cause of your problem.
2 They coax and model behavior change, leading by example, and nudging you in the right direction.

3   They have some knowledge in nutrition and can help you learn to cook if you don't know much (either as a professional expert or as someone who has gone through the same things as you). They coach you; that's because the food part is the hardest part to get right for your energy level.

4   They help you identify imbalances in your life and correct them, such as pointing out that you're eating too much junk or not getting enough sleep.

There are advantages to a one-on-one relationship, but if you have a couple of people in mind, that works too. These characteristics make for the best buddies when it comes to assisting you with your Do-Over and all of your wellness goals:

Positive and Fun. The main goal, of course, is to get you juiced, jazzed, and inspired about living a happy, energetic, and healthy life. (Yes, the main outcome of your Do-Over, in addition to a younger body and mind, will be more energy than you dreamed possible.) Ideally, you're going to want someone who has a smile-all-the-time personality, even when she's going through some trouble of her own. Think of those mirror neurons I just discussed. If you're around someone positive, you'll feed off that energy—and that will give you the power to get through tough times, make good decisions, and lead you to a younger RealAge (that is, being younger biologically than your calendar age) with more energy almost every day.

Not Afraid to Be Critical. Seems exactly the opposite of positive, huh? Actually, it's not. In fact, for a buddy, you want someone who is positive first and foremost but isn't afraid to tell you that you're slipping up; that you need to take a right turn instead of a left. In the process of making positive changes for your health, it's not always about what you want to hear but also about what you need to hear. You may need that occasional smackdown. But you want someone who helps you get up after you fall and who helps you forgive yourself. All of us fail. And we have to get over the idea that making a mistake or two or three somehow means we should cash in our chips and call it a day. *Really*—stumbling doesn't mean anything. What *is* a big deal is to recognize the failure, with a smackdown if needed, and take new actions for the future. That's what your buddy keeps you focused on. That's why it can be a delicate process to find your perfect buddy. But I will say this: the more positive your buddy, the better you'll be able to accept criticism when it does come. So positivity and a willingness to be critical aren't mutually exclusive. They actually work perfectly together.

A Two-Way Street. It should go without saying, but you don't want to be the one doing all the talking. If you don't get feedback from your buddy, then it probably won't be very effective. I say this mostly for those of you who may use virtual buddies: Facebook friends, texting friends, people like that. Let's say you have a deal to text your buddy at the end of the day with the number of steps you took. This is a great way to stay accountable, and you don't need much in return, just a quick "Good job on those 10,067 steps." But if you text with no response day after day, the act of texting may help for a time, but after a while you'll lose steam on your Do-Over because you're not getting that all-important feedback. Though I believe strongly in virtual setups, this is the one big danger that comes with them: one of the buddies gets so wrapped up in what's happening in her real world that she loses commitment to the process.

Similar Goals or Places. While this relationship doesn't have to be as thought-out as one you'd consider on Match .com, you are hoping to have maximum compatibility. So ultimately, you should use as your buddy someone who can really relate to what you're going through—or better, someone who's going through the exact same thing you are, or is maybe just a few months ahead of you in her progress. The ability to connect through shared experiences is one of the most powerful parts of the buddy relationship. Let's say you're trying to lose fifty pounds: it may not make much sense to choose a buddy who's never had a weight problem. (The exception is a professional coach; some of our best coaches have always been thin but have helped people lose and sustain over twenty thousand pounds of weight loss.) A buddy who hasn't shared your experiences can empathize, for sure, but there might not be the level of understanding you could get from others. That said, I also do like the idea of someone who can serve as a role model for you, too. So picking someone who has succeeded on the same journey as you—even if their goals have already been accomplished— can work quite nicely as well.

A Lifelong Learner and Educator. There are lots of ways to show support: "You can do it!" "You're doing great!" "Don't worry, just get back at it tomorrow!" "Why in the world did you eat four hunks of banana bread?" Support is the backbone of the buddy system, but it shouldn't be the only kind of communication you exchange. I find that these relationships are the most beneficial when both parties can also exchange information and ideas about healthy recipes, exercise ideas, health news, and things along those lines. That doesn't mean you need to buy into every changing trend or story, but being able to talk to each other about what's happening in the area you're most concerned about will amp up the value and the benefits of the relationship.

Activity Partner. This isn't a must, especially for those of you with virtual buddies, but if your buddy is someone with whom you can do a daily or weekly activity—like daily walking or a weekly tennis match—then you add a layer of accountability that will help keep you motivated to stick to your goals and, ultimately, to change your bad habits into good ones.

#4 | Your Buddy Should Listen— and Encourage You to Be Honest and Vulnerable

I'm not going to sit here and suggest that you need to spend as much time picking your buddy as you would picking your spouse. But you can't just pick a buddy on a whim. Not any old friend or neighbor will do. Why? Because it has to be someone you can trust, who will keep what you tell her private—and someone with whom you will be completely honest. The whole buddy system and your Do-Over will probably not work if you're shady about what you say—that you took ten thousand steps when you really took only six thousand, or that you ate only a handful of chips when in reality you devoured four bags. So if you think you'd be tempted to lie to your buddy because you want to save face, or you fear that he'll judge you, or you're too embarrassed to tell her the truth, then that person is not the right choice for your buddy. You won't see the buddy benefits if you're not honest. Remember, this system works only if you're willing to be vulnerable—to show not only your successes but also your failures, because that's when you'll need your buddy the most.

Being honest allows your buddy to give you a kick in the pants if you need it, but in a nonjudgmental way—and with possible solutions. Here's one way to think about the kind of person you should approach about being your wellness partner. Pretend you ate a whole box of [insert favorite sin food here]. Now, your job is to tell your buddy what just happened. Think about a few people who you are considering asking to be your buddy and imagine what their reaction would be. The person who says, "You're an idiot with no willpower" is not a good buddy (unless that empowers you and gets you to sustain a change in behavior). The person who only says, "You're still wonderful!" is not a good buddy. The person who says, "Do you have any extras for me to eat?" is not a good buddy. The best buddy is one who will say something to the effect of: "Okay, don't beat yourself up for it, but it's my job to help get you back on track, because I care about you. So let's figure out what you can do next time you have the urge to splurge. How about we stick a bag of [*favorite healthy food*] in your fridge at all times, and the next time you want to gorge on cookie batter, you know you first have to eat the celery-carrot-hummus tray." Soon, your body will enjoy the celery-carrot-hummus tray. This feedback is the kind that a good buddy can provide. It's supportive and helpful but also honest—and not limited to the things that you want to hear.

So when thinking about who might make the best buddy for you, think about who has the greatest ability to listen and to help. This ability is one of the reasons why women tend to make the best buddies (sorry, guys), because they're often better at doing the two-step tango of listening and being supportive and helpful, rather than just being Mr. Fix-It: for example, "Just eat carrots instead!" This isn't helpful to someone who downed a pint of butter pecan. A better buddy can actually help you solve the problem yourself with tangible advice, such as the above technique of helping you identify the emergency foods that will work for you because you like them. If you give your buddy permission, she can be your mirror—and help you discover those feelings and triggers that you've trained your brain to react to with unhealthy or disempowering responses (gorging on coconut cream pie, for example). The buddy supports you in replacing those habits with the healthy practices that turn these moments into successes.

Choosing the right buddy can be tricky at times, because you certainly don't want to offend your closest friends, but sometimes the people closest to you just don't make the best buddies.

Also, you want to choose a buddy who won't sabotage your efforts to get your Do-Over. I know plenty of people who have friends who want to celebrate a ten-pound weight loss with chocolate cake. If you want to use rewards, and that can be a good tactic, you need to find rewards that will facilitate good behavior, not derail it. A reward could be, for instance, a new pair of running shoes. Once, I was working with a woman in her forties whose goal was to feel and look younger. So when we went out to celebrate her recent accomplishments with a healthy meal, I discreetly asked a server to card her. That, I guessed, was more meaningful to her than celebrating with a plate of nachos.

#5 | Don't Be Afraid of the Smackdown

In the above point, you'll see what I like in a buddy—and by extension, what I don't like. Basically, you don't want a buddy who doesn't reply, who doesn't care, and who doesn't help you follow your plan. But there's another quality that I look for, too: I don't want a buddy who bends too much. That is, one who accepts your excuses that "life got in the way." If your buddy bends too much, so will you. That's why you need to have somebody who can be fun but can also be tough when you need it: hugs most of the time, verbal smackdowns some of the time.

Why? Because I want you to be called out. And I want you to call out your buddy, too. The ones who fail with the buddy system are the ones who are afraid to challenge, afraid to call out errors, afraid to do a smackdown. It's the old tough-love philosophy. Now, I don't want you to be mean or abusive, and I don't expect you to endure that if you're on the receiving end. What I do want is for you to accept that there will be some bumps. Sometimes your buddy will carry you over them; sometimes your buddy will push you over them. And sometimes a buddy should look you square in the eye, grit her teeth, and muster a very stern warning that you, my friend, are stronger than a bowl of cookie dough.

The ideal smackdown goes something like this: "C'mon now. No excuses, You won't be able to take care of the ones you love if you can't take care of yourself, so when you take care of yourself, you're actually showing love for everyone around you. It's not selfish to care for yourself. It's what you're supposed to do to support those around you." Sometimes those are the words that need to be heard—and most of the time, they're easiest to accept when they come from someone close to you. For your buddy to make a difference for you, you have to be willing to accept—and even embrace—tough-to-take feedback.

I do online coaching, meaning that I respond to and serve as a buddy to as many as 150 people every night about their progress. Out of all of those people, I need to be harsh to probably a couple of them every night. To them, I will say, "This is serious. You are too important a person to do it this way." No, it may not be fun, and it may not feel "nice," but sometimes it's necessary—and, ultimately it's what's best for your buddy and for the people who love that person. Even in our executive health practice, we need to do smackdowns on stars or CEOs or even presidents. Some people are too imposing for one of us docs to do a smackdown alone, and so we team up: two docs together so the celebrity factor won't derail the straight talk. That's right, for us to help some stars get a Do-Over, we sometimes need a double buddy team. You may, too, if your one buddy isn't getting you to change behavior enough to hit your Do-Over goals.

I do think that there is a bit of an art to the smackdown—and you have to be willing to deliver and receive those tough-love messages. I remember the story of Rocco. He appeared on *The Dr. Oz Show* as a 270-pound diabetic who had multiple 97 percent blockages in more than one of his coronary arteries. When Dr. Oz told him that he had diabetes and a heart condition, Rocco started sweating so profusely that Dr. Oz called me during the commercial break and said he needed me to coach Rocco immediately. And so I did.

Rocco soon got his life on track—he wanted that Do-Over. He emailed me every day, and I checked in with him on his cell phone if he didn't. He couldn't get away from me. Rocco had amazing success early on; in fact, he lost weight too quickly: forty-three pounds in a month. He got rid of his diabetes, hypertension, and arthritis, and he reduced his coronary blockages. But Rocco would slip up from time to time, and I needed to step in there and give him stern talks. Every time I did, I circled back to the reason why he wanted to get healthy, why he wanted his Do-Over: because of his grandkids. So I asked him if he wanted his grandkids to see him in the casket. And I reminded him about the deeper *why* of this whole process. That *why* is the driver of healthy habits. It's what sustains motivation so your Do-Over is sustained. And that's what sometimes has to be the card that's called during tough talk. You need a buddy you can trust with your *why*, and a buddy who isn't afraid to use it.

When I talk to Rocco these days, he usually reminds me that he'd be dead by now if he didn't have the coaching to keep him going. That's great motivation for your coach to hear—it helps make the coach a better coach for you. And that's a fact that's true not just for Rocco but also for many of us. We need help to keep from falling back and needing a second Do-Over. Your buddy increases the odds that your first Do-Over will succeed, and be the only one you need to help you stay younger.

#6 | It's Okay to Pay to Find a Friend

Many of you will find your buddies right in your own world right now, and some of you may find them virtually—via such things as message boards of groups that have similar goals. But I don't want you to discount another option if it better suits your personality: a buddy in the form of some kind of professional coaching. That can be a trainer, a nutritionist, or even an online coaching group. (Mine is called

Enforcer eCoaching.) While this approach somewhat contradicts the principle of finding someone on the same plane as you, it does have other advantages. Some people, for example, simply respond better to the buddy system when they feel as if they're gaining not just support but also knowledge from a trained pro. Some people like the idea of trying to please the professional: "See, I can do it!" And some people really want assurance that they'll receive the support and information they need. (Paying for the service essentially does that.)

When I took the role of coach during the smoking-cessation program I headed, working one-on-one with all of the participants, I soon learned that my role was not to lead like a drill sergeant in the traditional sense—barking orders, delivering strategy, being in charge. I really was serving more as a friend—or a coach—someone to talk to, someone who could help, someone who was able to nudge people in the direction that they truly wanted to go.

Now, you do need some guidelines when trying to find someone. Do a little research to look into what kind of service they provide. Is it personal coaching? An automated reply when you log your data? Can your buddy be tough, supportive, and knowledgeable without being judgmental? Simply looking up online reviews of these services can provide some clues.

#7 | Your Buddy Helps You Build the Missing Piece

Let's spend a little time talking about stripping. (No, not that kind. I'll cover that in chapter 6.) I'm talking about stripping down the exteriors we all put up, and really trying to identify what we want out of life—and out of better health. Of course, there are a bazillion reasons why we're motivated to lose weight and get healthier, and I'm not here to guess what yours are or to tell you what you should think and feel. Some people want to buy smaller pants, some want to look better at work, some want to fit into their high school bathing suit, some want to run a marathon, some want to be healthy enough to travel the world. Your motivation is just that: yours.

That said, having worked with thousands and thousands of people, I feel I'm somewhat qualified to strip all of the motivations down to their core—what they're really all about. And if I had to boil down those findings, I'd break it down like this. Men, for the most part, are motivated by two things: being attractive to a potential or existing partner and wanting to be around long enough to have a meaningful relationship with their grandkids. For women, the drive to a better body, better memory, and better health is often about improving self-respect.

Whether their poor health is caused by simple sugars or cigarette smoke or some other harmful ingredient in their lives, many women lose self-respect when their health falters. This is due to a number of reasons, and suboptimal health does not have to equal poor self-esteem—often, if we really think about it, it is the negative meaning we add to our circumstances that makes them even more challenging. I've worked with women struggling in relationships with poor communication or where the woman may not be treated with respect, and that translates into low self-esteem, destructive behavior, even lower self-esteem, and so on and so on. (Many women of a certain era simply had relationships with their husbands in which the men did not treat women with respect.) So the quest for better health is about chipping away to reclaim that self-respect.

Recently, I had a woman come in for a medical appointment. At fifty-seven, she was intelligent and successful, but worried that her husband was going to run around with a younger woman. He always carried a picture of her from when she was twenty-eight years old. When she finally told him how she felt, he said to her, "You don't have to worry about me. You don't have any competition." She broke down and cried. Over the next three or four months, she took her health back in an impressive Do-Over—and her marriage improved. From her standpoint, she just needed a little validation from her husband, and it served as the impetus to get her going—and her whole life improved because of it. I find that many women are in this same situation; they're struggling with self-respect and working for a Do-Over to gain it back.

Now, I don't for a second want to say that self-respect is reached only at some finish line called X number of pounds. But taking the actions that bring you closer to your goals, whatever they are—in this case, improved health—will leave you feeling more confident, vital, and excited right now. And that is why the buddy element is so key to your getting and sustaining your Do-Over. That buddy provides validation, pushes you, supports you, and strips away all the BS that can bubble up from your thoughts and relationships.

That, in the end, is what allows you to focus on you.

Devotion to Motion

7 Things You Need to Know About Physical Activity

If you look at the landscape of today's exercise culture, you'll notice two extremes. On one side are the folks who won't, don't, or can't do any physical activity beyond the simple tasks of living. We all know that's a problem, because we've been barraged with the headlines about how lack of exercise is linked to everything from obesity and heart disease to diabetes and memory problems.

Simply, if you don't move around, you're not going to be around.

The other extreme is one that's really taken off over the last few years: the extreme exercisers. Those are the ones who do mud races, and adventures, and get thrills through activities that many folks would think are way too advanced for the general population. There's nothing wrong with that side of the spectrum for some people besides an elevated risk of injury, especially overuse injuries; too much exercise can actually overwhelm the system that helps heal you. While those people are indeed active and engaging in healthy behaviors, I do fear one thing: that the extreme side sends a message to the slothy side that exercise *has* to be that way to get your Do-Over. As in: if you can't make it across butter-greased monkey bars with zombies chasing after you, then heck, just sit back and have another couple of doughnuts.

The truth is that for optimum health—for weight control, for longevity, for keeping up your sex drive, for maintaining brain health, for feeling strong and happy—the exercise formula rests right in the middle with a big old dose of moderation. Or, rather: "I don't need extremes for maximum health—heck, in many cases, doing less gives me maximum benefits."

So here's your prescription for your Do-Over: a little regular physical activity, the key words being *little* and *regular.*

I get it: walking throughout the day isn't the sexy solution to your health problems, because, well, sometimes it feels more boring than reading an encyclopedia of instruction manuals (unless you are walking with your BFF or partner).

But just because an answer isn't splashy doesn't mean that it doesn't work: in this case, the simple answer is the one that does.

Simply, walk ten thousand steps a day. As we say, "10K a day, no excuses."

If you do, your destination will be the one that this book is all about: creating the life you want with the health you have to have, or getting that life-changing Do-Over. Science has found that this formula for walking not only helps you burn calories to help you lose weight, but also changes your body's chemistry to reverse some of the damage you may have done to it throughout your life.

What I like best about this prescription is that when you think of the Do-Over, you may assume that an overhaul has to be this monumental change in which you tornado through a phone booth to change from Clark Kent to Superman. But that's not what a Do-Over is about. You can change the functioning of your genes (remember the discussion of epigenetics in mini medical school) and erase all the years of damage that may have been done through inactivity, bad foods, high stress, and other life crushers with something as simple as taking a walk and making sure you stay active throughout the day.

It may seem that "just get out and walk" is the prescribed answer for the beginner primarily because it's just about the safest exercise we know, in that it confers benefits without putting undue stress on your body. While it's good beginners' advice, it's not advice only for beginners. It's advice for everyone—no matter your fitness level, and no matter whether you're at the start of your Do-Over, in the middle of it, or have taken all the right steps to be at the maintenance level of your new life. I still walk ten thousand steps just about every day. I do miss my target on rare days because of travel—most travel days I walk six thousand or seven thousand steps before getting to the airport, so I can hit the 10K every day. In fact, I'm writing this sentence on a plane after a nearly five-hour flight that still has another few minutes to go, but I have 11,986 steps on the day because I did a forty-eight-minute workout before my drive to the airport. In this chapter, I'll explain how simply walking 10K a day works for a number of reasons.

I fell into walking as a solution back in 1987. It's not as if I've been a walker all my life and wanted this to be an answer. In fact, I spent most of my life doing more vigorous workouts. I captained the US squash team in the forerunner to the Pan American Games, and spent lunch hours sprinting up and down the stairs in a skyscraper that left me with Niagara-worthy puddles of sweat. I loved those workouts— for the competition, the camaraderie, the rigor, and the way I felt while I was playing and afterward.

In 1987, as part of my job as the chair of anesthesia, critical care, and pain management at the University of Chicago, I was coaching people by phone to help them stop smoking. One part of this program involved having smokers walk thirty minutes a day above and beyond what they would normally cover in their everyday activities. I made them call me when they finished that thirty-minute walk. Now, there were lots of reasons why I had them do this—the least being the physical benefits. I had them do it because it was a habit that they could use to replace the smoking habit, and I made them call because of the buddy principles covered in the last chapter. I asked them to walk because it was easy, not daunting. There was no need to change clothes or shower afterward, and virtually everyone could do it. There are several reasons why the smoking-cessation program works (of more than 2,600 people who have completed it, an amazing 63.8 percent quit and stayed tobacco free at the seven-month mark); I think one of the big reasons why it works is because of the walking component. That helps participants not gain pounds as they regain their taste buds. And it reinforces to me why this notion of Do-Over is so important: we can take one of our world's most powerful addictions—nicotine and cigarette smoking—and then use something as simple as walking to squash the habit and reverse the direction of a person's future health.

After a few years of advocating ten thousand steps a day, the results were so astounding that I had to see if research had already been done that backed up the changes we were witnessing. I started to look at scientific studies to investigate whether hard data supported the positive results of walking on health. The early studies on activity came out of alumni studies from places like Harvard University and the University of Pennsylvania, and from the Cleveland Clinic, and the Cooper Clinic in Dallas. When I combined all the data, the answer showed that taking about ten thousand steps a day was key, for reasons I'll describe in a moment.

If you don't have a pedometer and have no idea how long ten thousand steps are, it equates to about five miles. But here's the thing: you don't have to get it all in one chunk, and not only by walking. You just have to make an effort to walk around more. For example, I hold walking meetings at work. I park the farthest I can from my office. I catch up on TV shows while walking on a treadmill. I even have a treadmill desk so I can email while walking at a slow pace, but hey, it's part of my job to walk the walk, so to speak. The point is that if you take thirty minutes a day and devote it to walking, and then just rethink how you spend some of your time, you can manage ten thousand steps every day.

I'm convinced—because of anecdotal evidence and the

hard data—that walking is one of nature's greatest preventive medicines. That 10K a day makes you age slower and develop fewer disabilities, all while giving you more energy every day. Even just looking at cultures that do a lot of walking—whether we're talking European cities or small country towns—shows that those places have low obesity rates and high longevity rates.

It's really the simplest thing you can do to improve your health, and as I'll explain, there's no reason why you can't start right now—even if you have to build up to those numbers. In this chapter, I'll discuss the "why" and "how" behind the magic walking cure, as well as go over some of the fundamental principles on how other forms of physical activity can improve your life.

#1 | Ten Thousand Steps Is *the* Magic Number—and You Can Get There

One of the most memorable families I have ever worked with was a group of three women from three generations: the daughter, the mother, and the grandmother. They all had health problems, including obesity and diabetes. As part of my work as the Enforcer for *The Dr. Oz Show*, I met with them to talk about strategies that could help the three women reverse their conditions. Obviously, one of my prescriptions was to take ten thousand steps a day. The problem was that Grandma was in a wheelchair. She was obese, had diabetes as well as arthritis, and the only time she ever walked was when she went to the bathroom.

No way could she walk ten thousand steps, she told me. We bought her a pedometer, and I asked her to do me a favor: "Just email me how many steps you take every day. Don't worry about the ten thousand; just write me how many you do take." She sent that email three days later, telling me her number: sixty-four.

Sixty-four steps a day.

What she did next changed the course of her life. I asked if she could now do me another favor: just add a few steps every day. "Don't think about ten thousand. Just never take fewer steps today than you took yesterday." She agreed, and off she went. Over the next several years, she increased her step total every day and eventually made it to ten thousand steps. She got rid of her wheelchair after two years, and then her walker after that. All told, she lost forty pounds, controlled her diabetes better, and virtually eliminated her arthritis. She got her Do-Over.

My point is one I'm sure you already surmised: if she can do it—starting from simply walking enough to go to the bathroom—then anyone can. I love her story not only because of the outcomes but also because it's an example of how taking small steps can lead to bigger goals. I'm sure she never thought she'd be able to take ten thousand steps a day, just as I'm sure she probably thought she was going to be confined to a wheelchair her entire life. Neither turned out to be true. And besides making changes in her diet and doing other things you'll learn in this book, she got there one step at a time.

Now, I'd expect you'd be curious about the reason why 10,000 steps is the magic number. Did I just pick 10K a day because it was a round number, or because it sounded better than 9,437, or because, hey, it's as random as the Powerball numbers, and this is just what stuck?

I wish science knew the exact answer as to why 10,000 works, but what we do know is this: ten thousand seems to be the minimum number that provides the most health benefit. In fact, 10K a day breaks down insulin resistance much better than 8K, and 12K doesn't help more than 10K does. That is, 10K gets you more health benefits than eight thousand steps, and doing twelve thousand steps doesn't get you any more health benefits than doing ten thousand (yes, you may get more fit, but your health doesn't get better for the long term). So 10K a day is really the sweet spot where people lose weight and gain control of diabetes (and even reverse it).

Why is that important? Because insulin resistance is a big health concern. Refresher from our mini medical school: when you eat food, it turns into glucose—basically the sugar that's used for energy throughout your body. Glucose gives energy to all of your organs so that they can continue functioning, and you can continue living. When glucose enters your bloodstream, it sends a signal to your pancreas to secrete insulin. This hormone works like a delivery service—when functioning normally, insulin is that FedEx delivery vehicle we talked about in mini med that delivers glucose from your blood into the cells of all your organs and systems. But when there's insulin resistance, your body can't keep up—and you end up with a whole bunch of glucose floating around in your blood with no place to go. That's what turns to fat. In

the meantime, that excess sugar in your bloodstream damages your tissues (like in your artery walls) and renders them
less functional. Plus, all that excess sugar does a host of other
things to put you at risk for health problems, and makes you
feel tired. So stopping this cycle of insulin resistance is key to
getting your body working more efficiently, storing less fat,
decreasing the problems associated with obesity, and getting
your Do-Over.

Some of that comes with diet, no doubt (see page 147),
and some with managing stress (see page 225). But walking those ten thousand steps is part of the equation, because
it's the limit at which insulin resistance seems to decrease
substantially, allowing you to reverse the cycle. Because it's
such a simple strategy with such major health benefits, 10K
a day is the first thing I prescribe my patients and the people
I coach or am a buddy to—for weight loss; for smoking
cessation; for diabetes control; for blood pressure control;
for decreasing the risks of heart disease, stroke, and certain
cancers; for treating immune-related issues; for better sex; for
better kidney, liver, and lung function; for greater resiliency
in the face of stress; for better sleep—in fact, for just about
everything you need for your Do-Over.

In addition, walking (and exercise in general) can increase
the size of your brain's memory center, the hippocampus, by
up to 2 percent in a year (the only part of the human body
where size really matters). But stay on the couch, and this
key region may shrink by as much as 1.5 percent per year,
adding to memory lapses and fuzzy thinking. One reason?
Exercise increases levels of brain-derived neurotrophic factor (BDNF), a "brain fertilizer" that helps you grow those

new cells and encourages better memory formation. You don't have to be a race walker to get more brainpower, but it helps. The people studied in this research who got their brain's hippocampus measured via a magnetic resonance imaging (MRI) scan started out walking just ten to fifteen minutes at a stretch, building up slowly.

And I probably don't need to even tell you what a great stress reliever walking can be. Your body is hardwired to spring into action when stress hits. Any threat—an oncoming truck or an upcoming tax audit—sends your nervous system into overdrive. As you probably remember from the mini med course, it's called the fight-or-flight response, and it floods your system with stress hormones, which gear up your body to either take action or take off. But if the stress in your life never seems to let up, those hormones do more harm than good. Your muscles stay tense, your blood pressure goes up, your whole body is constantly poised for a fight, and the anxiety wears you down. You actually become exhausted by that constant stress. As little as twenty to thirty minutes a day of walking, seven days a week, reduces anxiety. Researchers recently stated that physical activity might be the wisest of man's natural antidepressants: it's a cheap, safe, fast alternative to drugs that act on the brain's neurotransmitters to improve your mood. Drugs usually take six weeks to start working; a walk, twenty minutes.

A big study from Harvard in 2010 looked at more than thirteen thousand women to see who reached or passed age seventy in "super healthful" condition: no cancer, diabetes, heart attacks, bypass graft surgery, congestive heart failure, stroke, kidney failure, chronic obstructive pulmonary disease, Parkinson's disease, cognitive impairment, or physical or mental health limitations. What these super healthy ones had in common was physical activity. Those who did the most activity in their sixties (and that was nearly 10K a day, not even more than that) were roughly twice as likely to be super healthful after age seventy as people who did the least activity. And get this: walking is enough to bring on the benefits.

If you're not convinced by now, just do this: make a commitment to try it for thirty days. Every day, do what you can to get in those steps. Will you lose fifty pounds in that time? Of course not. Will you resolve all of your health problems? No, biology does take a little more time than that. But I guarantee that you will feel better, feel stronger, be more motivated, lose a few pounds, decrease your blood pressure, and create new habits that will provide the foundation to make all of the changes you want in your life.

#2 | It Still Counts if You Substitute Other Activities for Walking

You already know what I think about walking; it's probably the closest thing you have to a cure-all. So I'd love for you to get in those ten thousand steps every day, even if you do like to include other exercises or activities in your day or week. And if you can't, it's okay to substitute other activity for some of the steps. (This is where data tracking becomes especially important.) The general rule is that one minute of moderate activity equals a hundred steps. If you do twenty minutes of moderate swimming, you can count that as two thousand steps. Now, one minute of intense activity can count as two hundred steps, but no cheating, please—that intensity has to be off the charts if you want to count it for two hundred. To be safe, just use the 100 figure for other activities you're doing. For more specific examples, follow this chart:

Activity	Intensity	Steps Equivalent per Minute
Swimming	Hard	200
	Moderate	160
	Easy	80
Biking	Hard	200
	Moderate	160
	Easy	30
Roller skating/Blading	Hard	140
Handball		260
Jumping rope	Fast	260
	Moderate	200
Racquetball		130
Squash singles		260
Squash doubles		100
Tennis singles		220
Tennis doubles		100
Gardening		40 to 80
Water aerobics		130

You'll note, of course, that activities less intense than moderate-paced walking tally fewer than a hundred steps a minute.

So feel free to sub in any exercises you like, though I do recommend that you still try to get in those 10K steps every day—preferably outdoors if you can. Why? For several reasons:

1 You'll burn a few extra calories. Credit wind resistance, having to dodge people/potholes/puddles, going up and down slopes. Real hills make a bigger difference (and firm your tush).

2 You'll like *you* more. Self-esteem jumps from all kinds of "green exercise," aka outdoor activities: hiking, biking, surfing, striding around the neighborhood.

3 You'll think better. Just ninety days of moderate walking boosts blood flow to your brain by 15 percent. (Can you say "Smarter"?)

4 You'll have fun. The people, pet, and baby watching is better than most TV.

5 You'll get lucky. Whether you're looking for love, work, or new ideas for the front door, leaving home helps you find it.

One very important thing to note: exercise is not an excuse for eating more. Many people justify overeating with the fact that they sweated around in some activity for twenty minutes or so. It is very, very easy to outeat your activity, because in the grand equation between how much you burn and how much you eat, the average person will never be able to outburn a bad diet. (Even elite athletes have to deal with this reality.)

#3 | Create This Good Habit to Wipe Out the Bad Ones

Very often, in the business of changing health habits, you'll find that the person in question might have an Achilles' heel when it comes to food—that one thing you're just addicted to, or love so much that you can't picture yourself going a day without. I think part of this stems from our new consumerism, where there's a coffee shop on every corner bursting with sugar-laden, caffeine-infused drinks that market themselves as pick-me-ups but really only bring you down an hour or two later. These habits or addictions can be just as hard to stop as smoking. Research at Yale University has shown that sugar, fat, and salt are all addicting, and together (think Bloomin' Onions or Buffalo wings) they can be as addicting as heroin or cocaine, at least in animal models of addiction (and you and I are animals). Especially when it comes to food, there are so many choices, so many traps, and so many ways that we can be tempted.

This is one of the reasons walking is so effective: it helps you beat that addiction. Take the case of one of my patients, who is trying to eliminate soda. He drank three large cans or bottles a day, which comes to more than 500 calories of straight sugar. Those were 500 empty calories, destructive and highly addictive—not just because of the chemical addiction but also because of the behavioral addiction of having to have that soda at certain times of the day. But what would happen if he could eliminate those 500 calories? Over a week's time, that's 3,500 calories (the equivalent of one pound of human fat) that he'd automatically not have to carry. Most people will find that if they can eliminate soda or the equivalent sugary drink, the weight will just start melting off. But knowing that and doing that are two different things.

You undoubtedly can guess how this patient is beating the habit: by walking. The way he's doing it is by challenging himself to soda-free streaks. He sees how many days in a row he can go without a soda. One week, he did three days. Another week, four days. He's gradually building up. As of this writing, his record is seventeen weeks without a soda. He handles the cravings by walking. If he feels a headache coming on or really wants to reach for a soda, he takes a walk and drinks a glass of water. Not only does it help him get in those ten thousand steps, but it also allows him to resist the momentary temptation. More importantly, he's creating a new habit that can sub in for the old one. Behavior experts will tell you that when it comes to weight loss or health changes, the biggest difficulty lies in having to give up things, and our brain doesn't like to lose. Stressed? Your brain wants action. You may have trained your brain that the action to take is to grab whatever item is your particular Achilles' heel. The real key to handling those temptations is to make sure you require your brain to take different actions. In this case, when you feel temptation coming on, walking is the signal to do something—and satisfies your brain's need for taking action. And that's not even counting all the physical benefits that take place. It's a double bonus in that you not only avoid the bad stuff but also get the good stuff in at the same time.

I would encourage you to take the same tactic. Identify

what you think is your biggest dietary downfall and give yourself a prescription. For example, every time you're tempted to tear open a bag of chips, walk for five minutes, do five push-ups, or eat six nuts (or do all three!). Then ask yourself if you still need those chips. More often than not, you won't. You can, of course, create your own Rx for whatever your temptation is, but definitely include some walking—even if it's a small number of steps or minutes. In no time, your life-damaging habits will morph into gimme-that-Do-Over ones.

#4 | Ignoring Resistance Training Is Ignoring Your Health

If you look at the course of history, the physical fitness trends are merely a blip on the timeline. Your ancestors got their physical activity simply by living—whether it was through farming, or walking into town, or running from lions, or doing any number of things they had to do in the preautomobile ages. In the last four or five decades, we've witnessed repeated generations of fitness crazes packed into just a few years. What's in and what's out has all changed quite a bit. There was a time, for instance, when people thought that training with dumbbells or barbells should be reserved only for body-builders; not even football or basketball players were allowed in the weight room. Many people, especially women, shied away from weights because they thought they'd beef up like a slab of cattle and, why, no, they didn't want to have muscle exploding from every part of their bodies.

While weights can certainly help you get bigger and stronger in that sense, I'm happy to say that the tide has turned, and working out with weights is no longer looked at with scorn or as something that only specific athletes should use. We're not all the way there yet, but more and more experts and folks in the media acknowledge that one of the secrets to a healthier body is doing some sort of resistance training, in which you move some kind of weight (even your body) against gravity to put your muscles under tension, as opposed to cardiovascular exercises such as running or swimming that are more to work your heart. To be fair, weight exercises can be cardiovascular, and cardiovascular exercise does involve muscles other than your heart muscles. But moving a weight against gravity is almost always how resistance is separated from cardio—or how they're traditionally distinguished.

There are a couple reasons why it's important to supplement your walking routine with some resistance training. And by "some," I mean a short routine twice a week to get maximum health benefit for your Do-Over. That is what I do. Here's why: when you do resistance training, you're breaking down muscle fibers. In the days that follow, the fibers rebuild the muscle stronger in anticipation of the next time you try to break them down. So over time, you're adding muscle to your body. Why do you need muscle? For one, when you add muscle, you're better able to protect your joints when you walk or perform other cardiovascular activity. Resistance exercises for the muscles above and below your knee, for example, are the best way to prevent and maybe even quiet the symptoms of knee arthritis. That's because your muscles can absorb some of the tension that's placed on your body during that activity. They act as shock absorbers. More muscle means fewer injuries, which means you're more likely to stick to your routine and stay healthy. (If you do cardio exercise before and without building up some muscle, you increase your risk of injury and increase the chance that you'll get to meet one or more orthopedic surgeons.)

Second, more muscle is actually better at burning calories. That is, your body chews up calories you ingest to maintain muscle mass, whereas it takes very few calories to maintain fat. So you burn more of the calories you consume if you can send those calories to be burned up by muscle, rather than to slosh around and add even more fat.

Third, building muscle seems to help break insulin resistance, just as walking ten thousand steps does. So by improving the process of insulin delivering glucose to your body's cells, you're decreasing the potential damage that glucose can do to your genes, your proteins, and your circulatory system, and the chances that you'll store fat that causes inflammation.

Fourth, resistance and cardio training builds up brain cells and connections, which are the greatest users of sugar in your body. Building a bigger brain with more brain connections is a great way to stay thin.

Let me make clear for those who are still skeptical: there is no indication you will sprout bodybuilder muscles doing a low-maintenance yet still challenging resistance workout. To add that kind of bulk takes lifting very heavy weights and feeding those muscles with lots of protein.

Best of all, you don't need to join a gym or invest in any fancy equipment to do a resistance workout. Here are my recommendations:

◆ You can use anything. To put your muscles under some type of resistance requires pushing or pulling some weight—that's where the tension is created, and that's where the process of growing muscle begins. But here's the greatest thing: there are a million different ways to do that. You can do it with traditional methods, like barbells, dumbbells, and exercise machines you'd find at the gym. You can do it with medicine balls. You can do it with resistance bands, which are small and light enough to pack so that you can have your own gym-on-the-go. You can do it with household items such as unopened cans of soup, jugs of water, bags of potting soil, broomsticks, and many other things that can double as equipment. You can also do it with your own body weight. Yes, squatting in place is a form of resistance exercise, as are push-ups. (One of our coaches once even saw a man working out with free weights in the exercise aisle at Walmart, and that was the moment she thought, "Wow, no excuses indeed!") What's all this mean? That there's really no excuse for not incorporating some resistance work every week. It doesn't have to cost anything, and you don't need to use a lot of weight, but you do need to do something.

◆ You need to do it only two days a week, for about fifteen to twenty minutes each session. A short routine just twice a week will give you the benefits of adding muscle. While there may be some advantages to doing it more often (though certainly no more than three or four times a week, since muscle grows and strengthens during rest periods), for the purposes of health and longevity, twice a week is a good number. That's what I do, except when I'm on vacation and have a little more time. Then I do resistance activities every other day.

◆ Work your entire body. To get the most benefit, you should aim to do exercises that work your largest muscle groups, such as those in your legs and back, as well as all the muscles in your core. The core consists of the abdominal muscles, as well as those in your hips and especially your butt. Strengthening your core isn't about burning fat, it's about providing a sort of anatomical back brace—to improve your posture, prevent injury, and keep your back strong while navigating life's tricky spots. A strong core may help keep you safe if you slip on the ice—not because a six-pack of abs can break a fall, but because a strong core may help you keep your balance so that you don't land nose-first on the sidewalk.

◆ Don't ignore your hands. Building hand strength in midlife protects you from inability to do activities of daily life, like dressing, and mobility problems later on and keeps you active longer. It's also critical to walking the dog, carrying groceries, opening paint, rearranging furniture. To do it, you can pop bubble wrap, play with clay, squeeze a ball, or even just gently push against a wall (a stretch that will help prevent carpal tunnel syndrome, a condition that develops when you overuse the muscles in your hands and forearms, especially from being on the computer a lot).

◆ Don't carry weights while walking. You need to see your hands when lifting weights to not risk injury to the muscles and tendons that make up the rotator cuff in your shoulder. When you get tired or start focusing on dodging potholes, you forget about proper technique with those weights and increase your odds of meeting someone specializing in rotator-cuff rehabilitation.

◆ You can create your own routine. There are lots of resources to help you put together a regimen that works for you, and I encourage you to try different ones and to make a conscious effort to mix things up, to keep yourself motivated and to challenge your muscles in different ways. Just keep in mind to work your upper body, lower body, and that all-important core. If you need a kick-start, you can do the routine outlined below, which is the one I do twice a week. It'll provide you a solid foundation for learning about resistance training, allowing you to move into different or more advanced moves as you get stronger. Many of these moves include a weight-free workout option if you don't have any equipment but want to get started.

Strength Training Guidelines

Do each move for about eight to twelve repetitions. Do not lock your arms or legs, and make sure to keep your abdominals sucked in tight. Don't forget to breathe: exhale when you're exerting the most force (either pushing or pulling); inhale when gravity is doing the work to return to starting position. Especially at the beginning, choose a weight that's light enough, and use that until you can do twelve repetitions with no problem.

How do you know when you're ready to add weight? If you can do an exercise more than twelve times without feeling fatigued in the muscle area you're working, it's time to graduate to a higher weight. But go slowly and use perfect form. If you can't perform that move at least eight times, you need lighter weight.

The Do-Over Weights Workout 1
(from *YOU: The Owner's Manual*)

I do this routine once a week.

SQUATS
(Strengthens legs and butt)

Stand with your feet a little wider than shoulder-width apart and with your hands by your side. Without curling your back, squat down to the point where your thighs are approximately parallel to the floor (or before that—higher up—if you have knee or lower-back pain). Pause, and then rise up to the original standing position. Look straight ahead with your body facing forward throughout the movement. When you get strong enough, you can hold weights or soup cans in your hands.

LUNGES
(Strengthens legs and butt)

Stand with your feet shoulder-width apart and with your hands on your hips (or holding dumbbells). Take a long step forward with your left foot. Bend your left knee so that your thigh is parallel to the floor (or before parallel—higher up— if you have knee or lower-back pain). Make sure your knee does not extend past your toes. Pause, and then step back to the original standing position. Repeat by stepping forward with your right foot. Keep alternating until you reach eight to twelve repetitions on each side. When you get strong enough, you can hold weights or soup cans in your hands.

BENT-OVER BACK ROWS
(Strengthens back)

Stand next to a weight bench or a sturdy chair or some kind of park bench—almost anything works. Put your right knee on the bench and hold a dumbbell or a can of soup in the left hand. With your right hand resting on the bench, bend over so that your back is about parallel to the ground. Keep your left arm straight down so the dumbbell dangles toward the floor. Using your back muscles, pull the dumbbell up while slightly skimming your elbow against your side and lifting your weight to your chest. Pause, and then lower it, and repeat eight to twelve times. Then switch sides. Do equal number of repetitions on each side.

ONE-LEG CALF LIFT
(Strengthens calves)

Stand with the ball of your left foot near the edge of a stair. Hold a weight in your left hand and use your right hand to balance yourself against a wall or stable chair. Lift your right foot so that it hangs relaxed near your left ankle. Lower your left heel as far off the stair as you can comfortably. Keeping your knee straight, use your calf muscle to press yourself up on your toes as high as you can. Repeat eight to twelve times. Do an equal number of repetitions on both sides.

PUSH-UPS
(Strengthens upper body)

Get in classic push-up position, with your hands and toes on the floor and your back straight. (Get on your knees if you can't do traditional push-ups.) Lower your body so that your chest just grazes the floor, and then push your body back up, keeping your back straight. Repeat eight to twelve times.

CRUNCH VARIATIONS
(Strengthens abdominals)

Lie on your back, with your knees bent and feet on the floor. Crunch your upper body up toward your knees, but no higher than about 45 degrees. Clasp your hands behind your head to support your neck. You can do many variations of the classic crunch, including holding a small weight at your chest or lifting your feet off the ground.

ARM AND LEG LIFTS
(Strengthens abdominals)

Place both hands and knees on the floor so that your arms and thighs are parallel to each other and perpendicular to the floor. Your knees should be directly under your hips, and your hands should be under your shoulders. Look to the floor, keeping your head in line with your spine. Lift your left arm and left leg slowly off the floor and extend them straight out so your arm, leg, and back are roughly in one line. Return slowly to the starting position. Then switch by raising your right arm and leg. Repeat on each side eight to twelve times.

The Do-Over Weights Workout 2
(from *YOU: The Owner's Manual*)

I do this routine once a week.

CHEST PRESS
(Strengthens chest)

With a dumbbell or other kind of weight in each hand, lie on the floor or a bench, holding the weights close to your chest. Press the weights straight up from your shoulders, with your palms facing each other or your toes, and bring the weights close together. Slowly lower them to the starting position. Repeat eight to twelve times.

BICEPS CURL
(Strengthens arms)

Stand or sit with your arms at your sides and your palms facing forward. Hold a dumbbell in each hand and bend your elbows slowly so that you move the weight to your shoulders, keeping your elbows at your side. Return them to the starting position, and do not rock the weights or your body to get them up. Repeat eight to twelve times.

STANDING SIDE LIFT
(Strengthens shoulders)

Stand with your feet shoulder-width apart and your knees and hips bent slightly. Holding a dumbbell in each hand, lean forward slightly from the hips and let your arms hang straight down, with your elbows bent and your palms facing each other. Pull your arms up and out to your sides, keeping your wrists straight and elbows slightly bent. Lift until your arms are almost parallel to the floor, and then return to the starting position. Repeat eight to twelve times.

ROTATOR-CUFF ROTATION
(Strengthens rotator cuff)

Lie on your side on a bench or the floor with a weight in your top hand. Bend your elbow at a 90-degree angle and hold your upper arm against the side of your body, with your forearm across your body. Lift the weight by rotating the top shoulder outward while keeping your upper arm against the side of your body. Lift until your forearm is almost perpendicular to the floor. Repeat eight to twelve times and then switch sides.

OVERHEAD PRESS
(Strengthens shoulders)

Sit on a bench or chair for back support. Hold a weight in each hand and lift them until your forearms are perpendicular to the ground, with the weights at shoulder level. With your palms facing forward, press the weights above you until they come together over your head, with your elbows bent just slightly. Repeat eight to twelve times.

#5 | Technology Is an Important Resource, but More Isn't Always Better

I know, I know: ten thousand steps seem like an awful lot, especially if you have to count them all. That's why the pedometer became perhaps one of the greatest prevention tools ever introduced into the market. No thinking, no fuss: just a quick setup to measure your average steps, and the pedometer does the work for you. Easy. Awesome. Effective.

These days, of course, there are numerous ways to count steps (or mileage or calories), and that's through higher-tech gadgets and do-it-yourself smartphone apps that attempt to make life even easier for the user. You do the work; it records the data. Again, there's lots of value to that. In fact, I use something called an Omron pedometer and also a Fitbit and a Garmin GPS, which are pedometers that count the number of horizontal and vertical steps I take. The latter two devices can even measure how much deep sleep I get. (I tend to lose mine—device, not sleep—so I have three or four on me at all times.) And I know plenty of folks who use their phone to record data. All of these tools can be effective to help you gain your Do-Over. In fact, research shows that self-monitoring is an effective form of motivation in itself; simply the act of tracking some kind of data gives people incentive to reach better numbers.

Some people are better than others about tracking. I have several patients who have tracked everything they eat, all of the steps they've walked every day, and every minute they've meditated for more than five years—nearly 1,900 days of meticulously recording data and emailing it to our system. (We, of course, served as a buddy and emailed encouragement and information back to motivate the process even more. After six months, most of the people we coach go to twice-a-week reporting to help sustain the process with their buddy, but these particular women sustained their change by sticking with daily reporting.) Through this practice, and obviously, healthier habits), all got Do-Overs. The woman I have coached the longest (but who is typical of those who take their Do-Over) made her diabetes and her hypertension vanish while losing 62 pounds (down from 208), and she discovered a newfound confidence and self-respect. Basically, tracking acts as its own buddy system—a way to stay accountable. Yes, it's usually tracking to a database, a piece of paper, or some hard drive or cloud. But it's still part of the motivation and accountability equation. That's not to say that data tracking will help you get healthier per se—it's the food choices and activities that will. But tracking keeps you motivated to make those smart food choices and get out there and walk.

There is one caveat to this whole self-monitoring, data-tracking issue. At some point during the day, you need to see the totals of what you have done. You don't have to obsess over them, and you don't have to beat yourself up over them, but you have to see them. What do I mean by that? Well, with all of this new technology, there are now forums and systems that tabulate your data for you—you just submit data with a click or a swipe and never have to see the accumulated totals unless you choose to. That is, maybe you never see how many steps you take by the end of the day, or maybe you never ever peek to see what your daily calorie total is. The technology is great in that it will run the numbers, add them up, and show you trends, but if you never bother to see what you did that day and each day—remember that accountability component—it doesn't do you any good in terms of motivating you to hit your goals. There's no feedback to tracking if you don't look at your totals each day; remember, 10K a day, no excuses. So make sure that whatever device you use, you don't overtech yourself to the point that you're not participating in the process. Add the numbers, see the numbers, be motivated by the numbers.

Now, I will also say that sophisticated analysis of numbers can play a very valuable role in some areas. For example, many people use numbers and data to optimize exceptional performance. That's a great thing, especially for elite athletes and those who make a living based on whether they're a quarter-second faster or slower than the next person. But the majority of us don't need the uberanalytics. For your Do-Over to optimal health, it's just the process of tracking—and the accountability that comes from doing so with a buddy—that matters.

One warning: don't rely on technology alone. Technology can backfire, and you don't want that to be an excuse for why you're not hitting your daily goal. Sometimes trackers are not accurate, especially when it comes to calorie burns and calorie counts, so there is a chance that error will lead to overeating when you think you've burned more than you have.

That said, there are two pieces of technology that I do think are essential: namely, a pedometer and a pair of quality shoes. I suggest buying two pedometer (in case you lose one; there's no excuse not to track your steps). And if you try to walk in ratty old shoes with no support, you're asking for an injury—which will derail your efforts to get healthy. Here are my favorite tech items:

♦ **Omron pedometer.** I go through two of these every year and one or two battery replacements, but I like these high-quality, cost-effective digital pedometers for accurately counting my steps. They're easy to set up and easy to use. I also like some other devices, such as the Fitbit, which track a lot of data. And GARMIN, Jawbone, and Microsoft all make nice wristband-style trackers that measure distance, steps, and calories burned. But these latter four choices require extra charging. I suggest you take some time to shop around, see what you like, what fits best with your lifestyle, and what will best keep you motivated. (Some models even buzz when you've been inactive for too long—a technological buddy!) For starters, just a simple but accurate count of steps is all you need to keep you true to the goal of ten thousand steps a day.

◆ **Cross-training shoes.** If you're going to do that much walking, you need a pair of shoes that provides the support you need. I recommend going to a specialty running/walking store that can help you find a shoe that's not only comfortable but also fits your foot and gait well. Shop in the late afternoon, after you've been on your feet for a good part of the day—your feet swell then, and that's when you want to have your shoes fitted. With so many choices, not just in style and color but also in function, it helps to have a pro work with you. If your shoe isn't the right one, you risk making your walk uncomfortable at best and injurious at worst. You may go through shoes fast—I need a new pair every three months—but the expenses on the front end of prevention are much easier to manage than expenses on the back end of treatment.

♦ **E-coaching.** If you can afford it and you have trouble finding a buddy who you work well with, it might be worth investing in some kind of online coaching. This technology allows you to maximize all of the benefits we talked about in the previous chapter, by logging your data and receiving education and feedback from someone who is very knowledgeable about nutrition, who understands how you're doing, and who can give you a kick in the pants when you need it.

♦ **Treadmill desk.** If money is no object (or if your company has a vested interest in its employees' health), maybe you can try one of these. It sure beats sitting all day, which leads to back pain and a host of other problems that stem from inactivity. I have one and find I can get in a lot of steps while doing some work: for example, I can write with a pen at 1.7 miles per hour and at a 2 degree incline. I can type on the computer at 1.8 mph and 2 degrees, read on computer or paper at 1.9 mph and 2 degrees, and take conference calls at 3.3 mph and 2 degrees. (Unless I'm talking: then it's 1.9 mph and 2 degrees.) If you do live at your desk, at least get up and walk around frequently (two minutes every thirty minutes seems to be key). This also keeps your head clear, and you never know what you'll see or learn: maybe some new office gossip, or maybe some innovative ideas will pop into your head as you move out of the borders of your work space. You can even get a portable headset if you're on the phone a lot. That way you can walk and talk.

#6 | If the Goal Is a Do-Over for Optimum Health, or Just Staying on Track for Optimum Health, Why Risk It with Lunacy?

I'm going to tell you a story that may inspire some of you and may frighten others. Caldwell Esselstyn Jr. won the gold medal in eight-man rowing in the 1956 Olympics. Ever since his competition days, he's been really into exercise and training. He loves it. He loves to compete, and he loves to work hard—no doubt from habits he formed as a young-ster and as part of the Yale University rowing team. Even at eighty-one years old today, he's in great shape. But Essy is a bit of a crazy man, too. He's had three major cycling accidents—each one taking a little bit out of him. Two were actually life threatening: In one, his wheel got caught in a branch and flipped him over. He was wearing a helmet, and luckily he was only a mile away from the hospital, where he underwent emergency brain surgery that saved his life.

Thirty-three months after that, Essy was out riding again. He was going down a hill very fast—cars were on one side of him and a mother with a baby stroller on the other. He spotted a rock in his path. He didn't want to hit the pedestrians, and he didn't want to go into traffic. So he took on the rock, flipped over again, and fractured his pelvis in more places than you can count on your fingers and toes. Despite the major damage, he recovered. And is back to cycling outdoors. (By the way, he still has all marbles intact, and while convalescing from that accident he wrote a landmark medical paper with his colleagues—I am one of them—on the 200 patients of whom 89 percent were adherent to his "Prevent and Reverse Heart Disease Diet.") I suggested to him that he should just set up a stationary bike, and he could get a computer program that allowed him to set up a screen from a cyclist's point of view to make it appear as if he were riding through beautiful vistas to simulate that feeling. It wasn't the same, he said. And while I agree that it's not the same, and I certainly admire Essy's passion and intensity, his story brings up a really important distinction to make when it comes to activity.

It's really vital to articulate your goals for your Do-Over at some point. If your goal is optimum health, then you should decide not to engage in high-risk activities that could derail you from reaching your main goal. Now, if your goal is adrenaline, that's fine. But I think you're reading this book because you want to live long, with vitality and spirit and energy and strength every day. And you're not going to have that if you're laid up with an acute or chronic injury.

Essy's example may be an extreme one, but I see this same sort of thing all the time. I have a friend, for example, who loves to play basketball with his friends, but he's already torn a calf muscle, and he pulls a muscle in his back or buttock nearly every game and sometimes can't even walk the next day. He likes the competition and the sweat, but he pays for it—and it ends up sidelining him from other activities that he enjoys too.

Now, I don't want you to give up activities you love, but I do have to challenge you to ask yourself: "Am I sure I love that activity so much that it's worth possibly being sidelined and not achieving my main goals?"

That's why I make a conscious decision to pick activities that I not only enjoy but also that have a low risk of injury. I want that strength and energy every day, and I don't want to creak and squeak because I rolled an ankle or broke a bone. I'm not suggesting that you live life scared. I just want you to make smart choices that minimize your risks while maximizing your joy. And joy is indeed a huge part of the equation: research from the University of New Hampshire shows that people who remembered something pleasant about an exercise session worked out up to 60 percent more often than those who remembered the negative feelings associated with their workouts. So that "no pain, no gain" mantra? It's not reality.

It is worth noting that "risk" isn't the same as "intensity." You can still engage in intense activity, and there are plenty of benefits to that kind of all-out effort (assuming you are in proper shape). High-intensity exercise raises your metabolic rate, even after you're finished. Perhaps more importantly, it is best at promoting positive changes in the brain as well. Specifically, studies have found that it helps regrow neurons that diminish the symptoms of the chronic progressive neurological disorder Parkinson's disease. That's the BDNF, or brain fertilizer, I mentioned earlier. More vigorous physical activity at any age increases your hippocampal size and your brain connections (whether or not you have Parkinson's). Exercising your leg and core muscles may work wonders for both your waist and your brain. Get your heart rate up to 85 percent of your age-adjusted maximum for twenty minutes three times a week, and you'll see the maximum benefit. (Here's the formula for determining your age adjusted maximum heart rate: 220 minus your age; for greater accuracy, subtract 64 percent of your age from 211.) If you are fifty-five, your maximum heart rate is about 220 minus 55, or 165. Fifteen percent of that is about twenty-five, so for optimum cardio you want to hit 140 beats a minute for 20 minutes three times a week with a couple of minutes of high intensity exercise (see below) for each twenty-minute period, if your doc says it is okay to do so.

High-intensity training, or interval training, has proved to be especially effective. As an example, you would swim, or walk, or run for one minute with a very hard effort. Next, move to an easy exercise for one to two minutes, to allow your body to recover, and then repeat the cycle several times. I like doing this in my own workouts a few times a week, be it on the treadmill or on a stationary bike that also works the arms.

#7 | You Can Outsmart Any Excuse

In my line of work, as you can imagine, I've heard just about every reason and excuse for why a person won't exercise:

"I'm hurt." "I have no energy." "I'm bored." "I don't want to put my body on display at the gym." "I'm busier than a dog with a caught squirrel and have no time to exercise." The craziest one I ever heard was the story of a man who used to run laps around the block to reach his 10K steps; he said he didn't want to run or to walk anymore because his wife, pregnant with their first child, was three months from her due date, and he didn't want to be too far away from her. (What's that cell phone in your pocket for?)

I should note that there does seem to be some genetic predisposition to enjoying exercise. Some recent studies of rats from the University of Missouri show that we may have genetic links toward activity, meaning that some of us could be predisposed to enjoying activity—though, as you know now, you don't have to be stuck with genetics that say you don't like exercise; you can find ways to enjoy it more.

I hope that by now you've seen ways to outfox those excuses, especially when it comes to walking. Think about it: walking is about the simplest and easiest exercise there is. You don't need to change clothes. You don't need to shower afterward. And unless you're a truck driver or in a job where you're strapped to a seat, you can find ways to get those steps in naturally. For example, I use a restroom at work that's not the closest one to my office. While on the treadmill, I catch up on reading or watching my second favorite TV show (*The Daily Show; Dr. Oz* is the favorite). I'm busy, too, but I let those numbers accumulate throughout the day. You can do the same. I also have a solution for just about any excuse you want to try on me:

Excuse	Solution
"It hurts to even walk."	You don't have to hit ten thousand the first time out. Just take a starting number and add a few steps every day. You'll eventually build up to that number. Walking actually has been shown to decrease inflammation and delay or even eliminate the need for knee replacement in people with osteoarthritis—the same holds true for the hip.
"The only time I am free is at night, and I'm just too exhausted by the time work and the family hangout are done."	Get in what you can during your workday: park farther away; get off the subway or bus one stop early and walk the rest of the way to work before you settle in. You'll find that these walks will increase your energy—and have more benefits in the long run.
"I don't want to spend money on a pedometer."	While I believe that a good pedometer is well worth the money, you can do approximation: a hundred steps equals one minute of walking. Just count your minutes.

Excuse	Solution
"I've got a cold."	Walking will help you prevent them. Every step you take mobilizes immune-system warriors that patrol your nose, throat, and lungs to take down invading cold and flu viruses. The benefit lasts for several hours after you take off your sneakers—which may be why (this is news) people who exercise five or more days a week have 46 percent fewer colds than those who work out once a week or less. When regularly active people do catch a cold, their symptoms (sneezing, congestion, coughing, dripping) are 41 percent less severe. But walking can be done with almost any cold. Just do it where you do not pass viruses to others.
"I want to lose weight before going out in public."	Walk in the privacy of your own home: buy a walking video, do circles in the house, yank the laundry off that dusty treadmill. Or pull on workout clothes you feel okay about, such as sweatpants and generous tops, and hike the neighborhood when few people are around. In a string of recent studies, overweight adults with good cardio fitness were less likely to die young than even unfit folks of *normal* weight.

Excuse	Solution
"My knee hurts."	Exercise itself won't increase your risk for developing arthritis. In fact, a moderately paced walk—or other low-impact activities such as swimming or using an elliptical trainer—plus light-weight strength training seem to keep the cushioning cartilage in your knee joints healthier.
"I'm pregnant."	A program geared to your fitness level can ease the baby-on-board effects such as backaches, constipation, and sleep problems. Junior benefits, too: exercising moms-to-be deliver babies with healthier birth weights, which lowers baby's risk for weight problems later on.
"I'm too stressed."	In a huge recent analysis, people who got physical for as little as thirty minutes a day cut their anxiety levels by almost a third, even if they were dealing with severe mind-body health stressors such as cancer. Male, female, young, old, doing moderate walks or sweaty, full-tilt workouts, it doesn't matter a hoot. You'll feel more at ease afterward.

Excuse	Solution
"It takes so much time to change, shower, and go to the gym."	That's another one of the many reasons why walking is so wonderful. No muss, no fuss, you can do it anywhere.
"I like to take a rest day."	We can agree on rest days for cardio and for resistance: three days a week max for each. But a rest day from 10K is not needed or beneficial.

Better Plate Than Ever

7 Things You Need to Know
About Nutrition

The world has plenty of famous threesomes: sci-fi fans may think of the original *Star Wars* trilogy. Music fans may immediately conjure up images of Destiny's Child or the Bee Gees. Baseball historians may think of Tinker to Evers to Chance, the Chicago Cubs' legendary double-play combination of the early twentieth century. That's not even mentioning the Stooges, the Musketeers, the little pigs, the Kardashian sisters, or a BLT. We're going to talk about the threesome that serves as the foundation for making sure your Do-Over is a success: the first three chapters of this book. In chapters 1 and 2, we talked about the importance of exercise and of a buddy. Chapter 3 addresses perhaps the most complex and difficult of the three core areas: navigating the world of nutrition.

In many cases, food is what got you into this spot of thinking that you needed a Do-Over. Too many bad meals, too many bad snacks, too many portions that resemble a

Nepalese mountain range added up over many years are the primary culprits that lead to weight gain, obesity, and problems associated with obesity, such as arthritis, cancer, diabetes, and heart disease. For many of you, it's the absolute hardest thing to change—because bad foods are addictive, they comfort us, they pleasure our tongues, and they can be easy to have, buy, and nuke. (A hot dog cooked in thirty-seven seconds is admittedly lower maintenance than a grilled salmon salad.)

This is why so much of what I talk about in this book comes down to a central theme: you must change your environment to increase your chances of having a successful Do-Over. Worry less about trying to resist banana cream pie and think more about not letting it in your house in the first place. Do that, and you'll set yourself up for success.

The reason why food is so dang important—and perhaps the most vulnerable stool leg in the trinity of food, exercise, and buddies—is that the fuel that you put into your body doesn't simply work for or against you based on its number of calories: food also causes chemical reactions that have a major effect on your genes and proteins. That's right. We've spent too many years focusing on calorie counts in food and not enough time thinking about the quality of our food. And when we talk about optimum health and gaining your health back from months, years, or decades of poor health and bad health choices, it's about changing the way your insides work—not necessarily how you look on the outside, although that will come as a side effect. So that's what this chapter is all about: I'm going to help you navigate all the nutritional information that's peppered at us constantly, so you can have the knowledge, tools, strategies, and motivation to make the changes that can change your body.

Even if you do know all the nuts and bolts (and by the way, nuts = good!), I'm going to take you through details of what works, what doesn't, and how you can make good nutrition happen. First, though, I want to give you a little perspective on how I became so passionate about nutrition. I think sometimes the perception is that we doctors who preach about good diets are robotic and soulless fruit fanatics who have programmed ourselves to never wade into the goo that is a cookies-and-cream monstrosity brownie sundae. Even though the practice-what-you-preach set does have better than average adherence to optimum nutrition, that doesn't mean we don't understand the suffering that so many face when trying to step away from the peach pie. And it doesn't mean that we don't have our own Achilles' heels that can trip us up. However, our job isn't just to teach you what works but also to make sensible eating simple and fun for you—the way we have in our own lives.

Up until about my thirteenth birthday, I was a chubby kid. Though I was active, I still carried some extra weight. I loved potatoes of any kind: fried, baked, mashed with garlic and butter. The more, the better. After I hit a growth spurt, I thinned out a bit and played more and more sports, my favorite being squash; little did I know that would become one of my favorite vegetables. In college, I was still thin, but I wasn't eating that well. That makes a vital point: just because you're thin doesn't mean that you're optimally healthy or not doing damage to your insides. In fact, because I was thin and active, I felt like I could eat anything. So I ate a lot of steak and a lot of simple carbohydrates. (Spaghetti with meat sauce became my favorite.) And I'd have at least a liter of regular (full sugar) soda a day. Once I got into medical school, my habits didn't get any better. For dinner, I'd eat a lot of red meat, still drink that soda, and have a baked potato smeared with butter. I didn't know any better. Heck, even in medical school, we didn't receive any nutrition training; yes, we had some guidance on vitamins and minerals, but we spent as much time on nutrition as art students spend on calculus. And we also had zippo instruction on how to cook or even how to use a knife, one of the keys to cooking and eating well. That also explains why so many doctors, especially of a certain generation, know only the basics or very little about nutrition. It simply wasn't part of our training. When I met the woman who would become my wife, Nancy, we would go out to eat a lot: fried chicken, biscuits, pizza, you name it. Only rarely did we go out and have healthy meals, like ones that would fall into a Mediterranean-type diet. I still ate a lot of red meat; in fact, when I was in Argentina to play squash in the forerunner to the Pan Am Games, that was just about all we had.

Then in the late 1980s, more and more research started coming out about saturated fats, trans fats, and simple carbohydrates, and their effects on heart disease, LDL (lousy) cholesterol, and inflammation. When we put all of this research together as part of the RealAge project, it became very clear what the primary food felons were:

1 Saturated fat
2 Trans fat

3 Simple sugars

4 Simple carbohydrates

5 Added syrups

In 1995 I decided to eliminate those felonious foods from my diet. That, I am sure, was the moment that my health, my body, and which of my genes were on changed for good. That's because, even though we didn't know it at the time, I was able to flip the switch on my genes so that my body functioned optimally. I got my Do-Over—and I didn't even know it.

Now, some people may think I live on the extreme side. (I've eaten only two ounces of red meat since 1995, and that's because I was the guest of honor at a famous person's home, and this individual made beef tenderloins for dinner; I felt it would be rude to refuse to eat the meal.) But I don't look at it that way. I look at my healthy eating the way I want you to try to do for yourself: I enjoy what I eat, and 99.9 percent of what I eat is good for me. I also look at my diet as an investment: an investment in high energy, good health, better sex, a sharper mind, stronger relationships, less stress, more productivity, more fun, and so many other benefits.

But don't just take my word for it. Take the word of Janelle. More than two years ago, her husband was diagnosed with a rare and aggressive form of cancer. They were told he had a 90 percent chance of dying from it within six months. Just a few months ago, she and her husband celebrated National Cancer Survivors Day—as well as the fact that Janelle reached her own goal of losing eighty-six pounds in one year. Last year she realized that to be a true caregiver, she needed to make her own health a priority. She started walking, accepted coaching, started logging every bite she ate, and changed everything, including giving up all five food felons, from fried food to sugar-laden drinks.

Today Janelle adds chia seeds and flaxseed to smoothies. She eats smaller and more frequent meals. She eats oatmeal for breakfast five days a week. She eats lots of vegetables. She orders foods without cheese or sour cream, and checks out menus online before going to a restaurant so that she knows in advance what to order.

Now her health problems are in remission (she had two gastrointestinal-related conditions), and she has set herself up to avoid so many other health problems because of the weight that she lost.

"I got a Do-Over," she told me. "This is the motto that I wrote down and taped to my bathroom mirror. It is the first thing I see every day."

We simply have two choices each day:

1. Make excuses

2. Make something happen.

The choice is yours. What will you choose today?

I chose and continue to choose to stop making excuses and to stop killing myself with a knife and fork.

And that's exactly what I want you to do: stop killing yourself with a knife and fork and spoon and gravy ladle and chocolate-stained fingers that "accidentally" took a deep dive into the Nutella. Enjoy and have fun with great food. In this chapter, I will outline how to do your food Do-Over, but the one thing I want you to keep in mind is that this battle isn't about outmuscling the Fritos with your willpower. It's all about changing your environments—whether eating in or eating out—so you don't even need willpower, so that your healthy choices are as automatic as the flip of a light switch. Here's how to get it all started—and change the way you eat (and live) forever:

#1 | Avoid the Five Food Felons

Anybody who knows me knows this: I almost always try to turn things around to say the positive rather than the negative. I'd rather say do than don't. I'd rather say can than can't. (I think of *can't* as a four-letter word; we didn't allow our children to say it ever.) I'd rather say yes than no. I'd rather say "Breathe free" than "Stop smoking." And I'd rather say, "Enjoy the ocean trout" than "Drop the bacon burger." But I'm going to make an exception as we start this chapter: I'm going to tell you what *not* to eat first. Why? Because the effects that these five felons have on your body are profound and lasting.

The biggest challenge facing most dieters is that they

think that nutrition is "Let's make a deal." As in, if you skip breakfast, you can eat pizza. Or if you eat veggies today, you can have Pop-Tarts tomorrow. If you have broccoli, you can pour a gallon's worth of melted cheese all over it. I'm sorry to tell you that your body doesn't work like a trade with the devil. There are no deals to be made, no souls to sell, no blackmail to engage in. Eat the wrong foods, and your body pays the consequences. And I must say that this isn't even about calories: you can't just "exercise off" a bad meal. While doing so may help control weight gain and can even help you lose weight, the calorie burn doesn't counteract the damage that these felons can do on the inside—and that's most important when it comes to overall health outcomes, longevity, staying disease free, feeling energetic, and enjoying a high quality of life no matter what your age.

Here's the reason: your genes make proteins that help your body function. For instance, hemoglobin (a protein) helps deliver oxygen and remove carbon dioxide from each cell. Most changes that are made to your proteins last the lifetime of that protein—as long as 180 days. That's the length of life of that protein in your body: 180 days! So when you eat ingredients and nutrients that are bad for you, their joy may last for an hour, but their ill effects on your body can last for six months. Even if you burn off the calories. Think about that: the joy of having the sugar in soda may last a few minutes but the damage that it does on the inside lasts for 180 days. Once those foods flip the switch, your eating a few handfuls of cauliflower can't flip them back. Here's more on that example: our friend hemoglobin, with a glucose molecule attached at the A1C position is hemoglobin A1C, which doesn't release oxygen to your tissues as efficiently; that changes the function of what goes on in your body. That's the real reason why you need to create behaviors that change your biological environment—and that's what allows your body to get into that Do-Over mode.

It will come as no surprise that many of these felonious ingredients are found in processed, artificial foods, but not all. And if you had to come up with an overarching principle when it comes to eating well, it would be that you should eat foods that are as close as possible to the way they're found on the earth. If they're not found on the earth, heck, then they're probably no good anyway. The felons:

1. Saturated Fats

Found in: red meats (yes, pork is a red meat), dairy (cheese, milk, ice cream), two-legged animal skin, and palm and coconut oils.

Saturated fats turn on the genes that cause obesity and inflammation, and promote cancer by turning off genes that kill cancer cells. While saturated fats have been up for some debate (namely, their role in cholesterol and heart disease), their devilish traits mainly come in the form of the obesity and inflammation-raising properties that they incite. Those lead to heart disease, impotence, memory loss, kidney disease, cancer, and promote diabetes. The debate about saturated fats—some saying there's no problem with them—comes from studies that essentially compare them to trans fats or data that ignore their long-term effects by their ability to create inflammation in your body and to change which of your genes are on or off. (See our Genetics 101 lesson in mini med for more on this.) So while saturated fats may look better compared with trans fats in terms of health outcomes, that doesn't make them healthy. They're the lesser of two evils. But something that causes obesity and inflammation in your body is still to be avoided. A side note: in the 1960s, a husband-and-wife research team had looked at margarine versus saturated fats. They thought margarine was going to have better health outcomes for people who substituted it for butter. Turned out, margarine, made with trans fats, was worse. The couple had staked their careers on their hypothesis, even promoting it in a book, and ended up committing suicide together by jumping off the Golden Gate Bridge because the results of their life's work were a sham. But the researchers didn't turn out to be wrong: saturated fats are still bad; just the substitute they chose was worse, so saturated fat did not look bad compared to trans fat. And what makes it worse is that saturated fats can be found in lots of different places (not just the meat and butter, where you may suspect them to be). They're found in flour-based desserts (which is the third biggest source of saturated fats, behind cheese and pizza), in chicken skin, and in creams and condiments. The problem is that these fats cause chemical reactions that hurt us. For example, they increase inflammation, promote obesity, and weaken immunity, and may increase some cancers. And new evidence suggests that saturated fats may promote fat storage around your belly; that's the most dangerous kind, because the toxins in fat are close to your vital organs.

BETTER PLATE THAN EVER

2. Trans Fats

Found in: lots of processed foods, such as chips, crackers, and cookies, as well as some vegetable margarines and foods fried in many oils.

Trans fats, an artificial form of fats made when hydrogen is added to fats to make products last longer, do the same kinds of damage that saturated fats do, as well as other forms of damage too. They raise bad cholesterol (LDL), lower good high-density-lipoprotein (HDL) cholesterol, and cause inflammation. Another thing trans fats can do is change the shape and structure of many of your receptors—they in essence poison the receptors that allow glucose to go inside your cells, in addition to damaging the receptor that allows your killer immune cells to dock and kill the cell—discombobulating your immune protection. These problems caused by trans fats can also contribute to greater arterial aging, heart disease, diabetes, and cancer.

Trans fats almost never occur naturally, with the exception of some milk and meat products; our bodies are not designed to metabolize them. *Always* avoid trans fats, even in small quantities. Stay tuned for how to identify if trans fats are in your food, even if they don't appear on the Nutrition Facts label.

3. Simple Sugars

Found in: juices, sodas, processed desserts, sauces, many packaged foods.

151

Simple sugars are often hidden on a package label, though they usually end in "-ose," like sucrose, dextrose, and maltose. They increase your blood sugar rapidly, and you remember from our discussion of fat storage and diabetes what happens when blood sugar levels rise rapidly—you're more prone to store fat, damage your arteries, and experience big swings in energy.

4. Simple Carbohydrates

Found in: white-flour foods such as bread, pancakes, rice, non–100 percent whole grain pasta.

These carbohydrates turn to sugar quickly in your body, as they are stripped of their whole-grain components. So these simple or "stripped" carbs are much less nutritious than 100 percent whole grain. Names such as enriched flour or semolina (a stripped pasta) are part of this category. And even foods that are labeled multigrain or a bajillion-grain something or other or similar wording are simple carbs. It's only 100 percent whole grain if the label uses "100 percent" phrasing.

5. Added Syrups

Found in: many processed foods.

These may seem healthier than added sugars, with names like organic cane syrup, or expeller pressed natural evaporated juice, or honey. But all of them, like the very common high fructose corn syrup, increase your blood sugar quickly and have the same effect on your body as simple sugars.

As you can see, three out of the five food felons fall into the category of excess sugar. No matter what form it takes, excess sugar in the bloodstream messes with the processes and substances that protect the integrity of your arteries. Excess sugar associates chemically with many of your proteins, causing them to be less effective. Case in point: the protein that helps the cells on the inside of your artery stick together is kind of like the grout holding bathroom tiles together. When excess sugar weakens the "protein grout" between the cells in your arteries, that allows blood pressure to chip away and damage your arteries, leading to plaque formation. This sugar also increases LDL (lousy) cholesterol, triglycerides (a type of fat in your blood), all resulting in an increased risk of heart disease. Not to mention that too much sugar wreaks havoc on the insulin transport system, which raises the risk of fat storage and diabetes, memory loss, impotence, wrinkles, and developing certain forms of cancer. And if that's not enough to make you arrest, ban, and imprison simple sugar now, do *not* turn to sugar after you develop cancer; simple sugar increases the malignancy—the badness and danger to your health—of that cancer.

You can see how and why all of these five food felons give you more of a Mess-Over than a Do-Over: they mess up critical chemical processes in your body. The other part of the equation that shouldn't be lost is that when you have an excess of these substances, it greatly increases the chances you'll store dangerous belly fat. This is especially true with saturated fats, as they turn on genes that promote storage of fat in your visceral, or belly, area.

Now, it should be noted that eating too much of anything (even good foods) can cause you to store fat, but the difference here is that these bad substances promote overeating, whereas good ingredients (listed below) help you stay full longer, satisfy you, and help prevent you from overeating. This is done primarily through the stimulation of the hormones leptin and ghrelin. When your ghrelin is increased (as it is when you eat these felons, especially certain artificially made syrups), you feel hungrier. And when your leptin is high, as it is when you eat foods such as healthy fats (avocados, walnuts, chia, salmon, olives, olive oil, anchovies, ocean trout) and fiber, your satisfaction is high, so you're less likely to overeat—and thus less likely to accumulate that damaging belly fat. Also, when you have sizable belly fat, that fat releases hormones that break down your brain's blood-brain barrier—a chemical fortress of sorts that keeps your brain healthy—to allow toxins to get into your brain. This barrier breakdown has been linked to memory rot and Alzheimer's disease.

#2 | Enjoy Eating!

If you ask me what my favorite meal is, I could rattle it off without hesitation: a big salad with mixed greens, lots of vegetables, a few walnuts, balsamic vinegar, and olive oil; mustard-crusted wild salmon; spinach and broccoli; and a glass of red wine as dessert. Love it. Actually, I have a variation of that quite a few times every week, I love it so much. There's not an ingredient in that meal that isn't good for me, but I love it not just for the health benefits but also because I find it irresistibly delicious.

And that brings us to the stigma we have to lift. This is what we have to change. And this is what I ask you to challenge yourself about: that good food has to taste bad. That's just plain wrong. While I know that nutrition can be the difficult part of the puzzle ("fat-free" on the label sounds as if that food should be healthy, but it's often not), I also know that it doesn't have to be. Learning the few basic tenets of healthy eating and cooking will serve as your foundation for establishing good habits—and for allowing yourself to have the creativity to experiment in all kinds of ways with those ingredients.

I've found that it takes a full three to five months to really "get it"—in terms of how to read food labels, identify which ingredients are good for you, experiment to find foods that you love, and know the pitfalls that are perpetuated by food marketers. One of the toughest things to "get" is that *cheese is not a vegetable*; it's made with saturated fats and milk proteins (which may also be hazardous, though the jury is out on that). Simply, it takes an awful lot of coaching and practice to make the switch from eating whatever you want to really understanding proper nutrition. Ironic story: I remember giving a talk to some of the best athletes in the world—Cirque du Soleil performers—and one of them came up to me afterward and said, "What do you mean cheese is bad?

I eat it all the time." She was Eastern European, and cheese was the inexpensive protein option in her country, she said. Here was somebody who needed her body performing at the optimum level for her career to do some of the craziest stunts in the world, and she didn't understand nutrition enough to allow her to be optimal for the long run. Maybe at the time it was no big deal because it wasn't affecting her performance, but those aging effects of saturated fats could catch up to her—maybe cutting her career short, or maybe putting her at risk for disease or other medical conditions. After I talked to her, she started eating nuts, seeds such as chia, and salmon burgers (which, when cut up in wedges, can be eaten almost like cheese), and really enjoyed her new choices.

Choose the Friendly Foods. Just as you should get to know your food felons, you should also know your friends: the foods that you want filling your plate. Know 'em, love 'em, eat 'em:

- ◆ *Fruits and Vegetables.* You can't go wrong in this category, whether it's berries, citrus fruits, cruciferous vegetables, or any others. Buy organic and frozen if fresh ones aren't available. Why organic? While some fruits and vegetables with thick skins—like avocados, cantaloupe, mangoes, pineapple—can be eaten safely, non-organic, thinner-skinned options such as berries, apples, and tomatoes absorb high concentrations of residual pesticides that carry their own slew of harmful metabolic impacts, especially for children and women in the potentially pregnant age group. Even with organic options, always be sure to wash your produce thoroughly in warm water.

Fruits and vegetables contain heart-healthy fiber, and they also contain the disease-fighting chemicals called polyphenols. Learn to cut them up quickly (see page 186) and prepare them with spices and herbs you love. Just keep trying them until you discover which flavors you find most delectable. (Cinnamon is always a good option.)

♦ **Lean Protein.** Protein in the form of fish, skinless chicken, and turkey, as well as beans and nuts, help build muscle (good for fat burning) and keep you satiated. However, you should avoid chicken and turkey deli meats, which usually are highly processed with harmful chemicals, in addition to red meat, including pork, and egg yolks. Red meat contains saturated fats and the amino acid carnitine, which (as well as lecithin and choline) changes the bacteria in your intestine. Yes, your poop has been formed by the bacteria in your gut that devote their lives to digesting what you eat. If you consume more than 100 grams of carnitine a week (about 4 ounces of red meat) or 1 egg yolk a week, or a combo, your bacteria change to produce inflammatory trimethylamine (TMA) or butyl betaine. Your liver turns these into inflammatory compounds like trimethylamine oxide (TMAO), which causes more havoc in your arteries than sugar or high blood pressure, and may be more likely to promote cancer than even cigarettes, and leads to kidney failure more predictably than even diabetes does.

◆ **Unsaturated Fats.** The healthiest fats are found in olives and olive oils, avocados, walnuts, chia and flax seeds, and wild salmon, ocean trout, anchovies, and a few other fish. Unsaturated fats work by helping to keep your arteries clear and inflammation down to a minimum. Many foods that carry unsaturated fats also carry some saturated fats, and that is okay; the point is to minimize the unhealthy sources of these nutrients and to choose foods with the most beneficial overall nutrient profile. In the world of fats, that is foods with zero trans fats, mostly unsaturated fats, and less than 4 grams of saturated fats per serving—like the aforementioned olive oil, walnuts, chia and flax, and fish. (When buying fish, choose those with low levels of the brain and nerve toxin mercury, such as wild salmon; avoid high-mercury fish like bluefin tuna, shark, swordfish, mackerel, and tilefish.)

◆ **100 Percent Whole Grains.** Grains that are completely unrefined, aka 100 percent whole grains, contain nutrients and fiber that help keep cholesterol down and digestive health up. They're slow to absorb, so you don't get that up-and-down addictive effect that you do from the release of sugar— causing you to want more sugar to maintain your energy level. They also help keep you full because of their high fiber, but you have to make sure that "100%" is marked somewhere on the label, or else you don't know how many refined carbs (which contain few or no nutrients) could be in the product. You can get these whole grains in breads and pasta. While they are fine to eat, I encourage you to prioritize these, in terms of volume, behind the other foods we've covered, and to eat grains that most resemble the form we find them in nature. I've discovered that after my generous dose of 100 percent whole grain oats in the morning, I don't need very much of these man-made whole grains throughout the day because of the nutrients delivered in protein, unsaturated fats, and fruits and vegetables. I recommend trying out some less common grains too. (See below for examples.)

It is worth noting that many people need or want to go gluten-free because of an allergy or intolerance to it. Gluten, found in wheat, rye, and barley, is the doughy protein that holds bread together. An abundance of whole grain options don't contain gluten, such as quinoa, amaranth, rice, buckwheat, and millet, and I encourage you to try them out regardless of your interest in going gluten-free. But be aware that many processed gluten-free products have all the felons of processed gluten-ful options and should be avoided. If you do need to go gluten-free, your best bet is to spend some time searching online for gluten-free products that are also felon-free. Note that you won't necessarily find gluten on an item's ingredients list. Check the label for under-the-radar, red-flag words such as *modified, hydrogenated, natural flavors,* and *less intense allergen.* And remember to avoid added or hidden sugars in the foods you choose that are gluten-free.

Automate Your Choices. Once you find foods and recipes that you love, have them a lot, especially when you are starting your Do-Over. For instance, eat the same delicious and healthy meals for breakfast and lunch five days a week. The more you can automate your actions, the easier it is to get into the rhythm of smart eating. This saves you from making bad decisions—and from falling for sinful temptations at times you may be especially hungry. Plan ahead, keep it simple, choose what you love, and pick some meals that you can keep consistent.

Think Small. While there is some debate today about the optimal size and frequency of meals, the research shows that eating large meals causes more damage to your body's energy factories, called mitochondria, than eating small meals does. This happens if the amount of sugar circulating in your bloodstream, or glucose load, exceeds what your cells can handle, as is common after a big meal. When that happens, your mitochondria can't convert the glucose to ATP (adenosine triphosphate) as well, and you start feeling like a ninety-year-old no matter what your age—or at least ten years older if you are already ninety! That excess load on your mitochondria is what creates damage and shrinkage of mitochondrial DNA over time. Less and/or less functional mitochondrial DNA means less energy for you. So it's better to eat smaller, more frequent meals throughout the day rather than gorge your bloodstream with all this excess glucose that will not only turn to fat but also damage your cells in the process, leading to a whole host of health issues.

All of your meals should be small. To help you get into the habit, use nine-inch plates instead of twelve-inchers. And if you can, decrease meal size throughout the day, with your larger meals coming at breakfast and lunch, and a smaller one toward the end of the day. Europeans do this— or at least they did—until we started exporting bad habits to them.

Redefine What Cheating Means. I know there are several popular diets that advocate a cheat meal or cheat day: a time when you ignore all the rules and eat whatever you want. While there may be some value in that approach in terms of giving you lasting motivation to do well the other 90 percent of the week, the fact is that when you eat one or more of the five food felons, you change the way your body works and how your genes and proteins function. You may be thin (this cheat strategy can help some folks lose weight and waist), but, following that cheat meal, your genes and proteins function as if you were very overweight. So does that mean you can never ever have a piece of red meat again? No. It just means that when you do deviate from the plan, serve very, very small portions—as I said, fewer than four ounces of red meat a week, for example, or just a spoonful or two of that sinful dessert. Cheat shouldn't mean gorge. Your body wants to give you a Do-Over if you let it. But if you make your system go haywire with a weekly dose of nasty nachos, you'll never be able to change gears completely and let your body recalibrate to the place it needs to be for optimum health. My guess is that when you do make these lasting changes, you won't even want to cheat with big-dose binges, because you'll have learned to love other foods—foods that work in your favor, not against it.

Make It Convenient—for You. I'd be a ding-dong if I thought I could tell every person how she should eat. I can tell you what to eat and why, but the *how* has to fit into your lifestyle, your schedule, your desires. So if it makes sense for you to go shopping on a Sunday and make a big batch of soup, a couple of meals, and lots of containers of raw veggies to have throughout the week, then do that. If you like to cook and experiment and dream up new recipes every night, then do that. If buying big bags of frozen berries is more convenient for you than trying to keep up with fresh ones, great! That's what I do with items like organic fruit, many veggies (like peas), and wild salmon burgers, and you lose no nutritional power by buying them frozen.

If your preference is to eat out, you can even do it that way, although, admittedly, this is a bit harder. You just have to know what to order and how to order. Consider yourself the CEO in each restaurant each time you eat out. For instance, you can order chicken fajitas—a very healthy meal—as long as you make sure to ask that it be cooked in olive oil, on corn tortillas (which are actually 100 percent whole grain), and served with extra veggies. Remember to skip the refried beans, which often contain added saturated animal fats. Or maybe you prefer to use a home-delivery prepared or nearly prepared meals service that provides you with a batch of meals ready to go with minimal preparation. My point: there are indeed lots of ways to fit healthy eating into your lifestyle. So don't let "Life got in the way" or "I'm too busy" be an excuse for why you can't (that four-letter word again) do it. You can. And you don't have to turn your life into an upside-down house of horrors to do so.

Why is this so necessary? It doesn't matter whether your goal is weight loss or curing a health problem, proper nutrition will get you there—for all the reasons outlined earlier. Eating these friendly foods allows your body's systems to function the way they're supposed to. Consider some of these personal stories, which help reinforce the data.

When David was thirty-eight, he had a heart attack. Five years later, he suffered a stroke. In both cases, he had confirmed blockages in his arteries, and ten years after his stroke, he underwent bypass surgery. Despite having undergone this major operation, medication, and some dietary changes, he was still eating sugar, fat, and meat—and he was still having daily chest pain, or angina. His doctor told him there was nothing more she could do for him. After seeing a TV show that outlined healthy dietary principles, David finally gave up sugar, simple carbs, and red meat. He occasionally ate salmon but mostly got his protein from vegetarian sources. He also started walking, gave up his occasional pipe, and was so worried about dying and leaving his wife alone that he started meditating, too. Within two weeks, David's chest pain during walking disappeared, and his erectile dysfunction resolved. After eighteen months, he had lost sixty-three pounds and felt (and was) so much healthier. Now, at seventy-nine years old, David is active, happy, and even bought a mobile home so that he and his wife can travel from Canada to Florida for the winter.

Jack, forty-four, had hyperlipidemia (high LDL cholesterol and high blood levels of triglycerides) as well as hypertension, which he tried to control with medications and by following the American Heart Association diet. His father, uncle, and several brothers had died at young ages from complications of cardiovascular disease. Recurrent chest pain and leg pain caused him to seek a Do-Over. He had already had his third heart operation to treat chest pain at that time, but he was an avid squash player, and new leg pain was inhibiting his ability to play. So he modified his diet to be felon-free by making sure to include only 100 percent whole grains, no saturated or trans fats or simple sugars, syrups or any non–100 percent whole grains, and adding lots of fruits, vegetables, whole grains, lean poultry and fish, and nuts. Within four months of starting the program, his leg pain while walking improved markedly, and his blood pressure normalized without medications over the next year. He was also able to play squash and golf without discomfort or pain. Two and a half years after having started the principles outlined in this Do-Over plan, Jack had lost thirty pounds. He now is seventy-two and has outlived all other men in his family.

Christine was diagnosed with type 2 diabetes in her early thirties, when she had two young children. She was overweight, on medication, and her sister and a brother had died of heart disease before their fiftieth birthdays. Soon after, she started experiencing chest pain, which turned out to be from the narrowing of her coronary arteries diagnosed by angiography X-rays. She took even more medication, and her docs warned that all four arteries had sustained severe damage. Christine opted for a Do-Over over surgery. Within six months of following this Do-Over plan, she lost thirty pounds, got her bloodwork in normal range with very few medications: only one cholesterol management drug, as compared with the four (for diabetes, high blood pressure, and cholesterol management) she was taking before.

All of these people—and these are simply three of many, many folks—got their Do-Over. They achieved it because they followed all of the principles outlined in this book, but mainly because they got their eating in order and let good foods work their magical biological powers to heal the body.

#3 | Have Regular Tasting Parties

Say the word *diet* or the phrase "eating right," and many people grunt and groan because they think their lives will be limited to bean sprouts, arugula, and two bites of grilled fish. That's when they think about how nice it would be to swan-dive into a pool of custard. But I see the words "eating right," and I see possibilities: all kinds of wonderful, great-tasting, youth-preserving foods, including guacamole, pizza, lasagna, fish tacos, you name it. The difference between what some see and what I see is the difference between being excited about eating healthy foods and thinking that eating healthy has to be a chore, has to be limiting, and has to be as bland as a piece of Styrofoam.

The truth is that the possibilities for delicious combos of healthy foods are infinite. The only thing holding you back, perhaps, is that you don't know how to make them, you don't know how they taste, and you rightfully don't want to spend the time or money on recipes that you may not like.

Here's how to beat that: start potluck parties with a small group of people who share the same goals and visions for optimum health as you. The deal: everybody brings a new healthful recipe using the guidelines above, avoiding the five food felons and using as many wholesome ingredients as needed to make the dish taste great. They can find recipes online or in a cookbook or make them up on their own, and then they bring the food (and the accompanying recipe) for everyone to share. Everyone rates the recipes for themselves and for the group. At the end of the night, you could have four or five new recipes to add to your arsenal of food preparation.

The reason that I love this approach is not only for the obvious opportunities to get ideas and expand your possibilities of healthful eating. But also, it deflates the argument that socializing has to entail gorging on pigs in a blanket and Buffalo wings. You can socialize while eating healthy foods and still have as much fun and get as much enjoyment from them as you do from fried mozzarella balls. (By the way, once you start eating real food, those mozzarella balls will taste like a vat of chemical soup.)

I do have some experience with this. As part of publishing *The RealAge Diet*, our team, including Donna Szymanski and Dr. John La Puma—who really taught me how to cook—created three hundred recipes. Before we included any of them in the book, I wanted many people to taste them and enjoy them again and again. And I wanted to make sure that I—a true kitchen amateur who before this could barely manage making toast—could make them in under thirty minutes. Every weekday for a year, we sampled six to twelve new recipes and invited eight to twelve guests to taste and rate them. Sometimes I'd just invite over random graduate students to try them. We tried (I made) each recipe multiple times. The dishes that were consistently rated "as good as great sex" or "would order again and pay for it" (a lesser rating) were tried on multiple groups of tasters. The dishes that got top scores time and again made it into the book. But that wasn't the point; the point was that it was great fun to learn cooking techniques, experiment with ingredients, and have others enjoy the tastings.

Nancy and I also have a New Year's Day party every year, and we invite guests to bring a recipe based on a certain theme (guacamole, for example), so we can see how people make it differently and enjoy new and healthy flavors. (For the record, we dip celery, not chips, into the guac.) This group-tasting concept works so well because it's fun and healthy, and because it always gives Nancy and me (as well as our guests) new ideas that we can incorporate into our own meal rotations at home.

You can do the tasting concept any way you want, but I like the idea of getting four or five like-minded couples or families or individuals into the club. You each take turns hosting and picking food themes, and each guest delivers a delicious dish for everyone to try. You can pick themes based on cultures (Mexican- or Italian-inspired, for example), ingredients (everyone must use a red pepper and a whole grain pasta or bread), colors (use a healthy red food)—anything. Or you can just make it a free-for-all and let everyone surprise one another with their creativity. These parties don't have to be centered around holidays or special occasions, but can be held monthly, like a book club. And the idea isn't to praise each dish but to be critical. "Good try, great idea, just doesn't work for me" is an appropriate comment. Or "Next time add some rosemary and more garlic and some roasted beets." Most importantly, the concept gets you over the thinking that healthy eating is limited. In this setting, you'll learn that it's exactly the opposite.

#4 | Learn to Read . . . Labels

I don't want your Do-Over to be about the blame game, with you blaming yourself for mistakes you made in the past, blaming your pants for not fitting the way they used to, blaming the world for your struggles that force you to the fridge. I'd rather focus on solutions than on problems, but I also understand that acknowledging what you're up against is part of figuring out the solution. And I will tell you this: one of your biggest enemies can be the food-marketing industry. These food manufacturers are in the business of enticing you into buying their products, and they'll use jargon to make you think their products are good for you. The lack of regulation on "implications" of words used in food marketing leaves you in the lurch. For example, a food might be fat-free, but that doesn't mean it's free of added sugar or carrageenan; it could even be a downright-horrible-for-your-health food, even though the fat-free label implies a certain wholesomeness. The same goes for other types of phrases, such as "all natural" and "healthy grains" and "fortified." All of those things can be absolutely true, but the rest of the product might consist of ingredients that are bad for you.

So the bottom line: you have to get beyond the hype and become an expert reader of food labels. The fine print is where you will learn which products are good for you and which ones contain the food felons. Reading the fine print arms you with information to make smart choices, to make decisions about what you eat, to make sure that the ingredients you're putting into your body are doing the right things for your proteins and your genes.

Now, I know it can be tricky. When some of the words sound like they're futuristic or foreign, you have no idea what they mean and whether they're good for you. Luckily, I'm not asking you to learn a dictionary's worth of new terms. I'm asking you to use clues to figure out your food labels. Here's what you need to know.

First, look at the back: the front contains the marketing; the back (the label) contains the facts. Buy on facts, not hype.

Quantity: generally, the fewer ingredients, the better.

Sugars: ingredients that end in -ose are variations of sugar. You want a total of 4 grams or less of added sugars in a realistic serving of any and all foods eaten within a one-hour period. (Unfortunately, quantities of added sugars aren't yet included on nutritional labels, but you can use the "sugars" value and a quick scan of the ingredients to guesstimate if a large volume of added sugars are present.) Added sugars are those sugars added to things as opposed to being in the whole unprocessed food, such as an apple. The problem is one of what raises your blood sugar. Soon you will be able to wear a device that measures your minute-to-minute blood sugar and can gauge your food choices by that number. Until then, just say NO to the felons.

Carbohydrates: if it is refined or enriched, reject it.

Syrup: if you see the word *syrup* in any shape or form, run.

Protein: don't worry about limits here. It is good for you, and as long as protein comes from sources without significant levels of saturated fat (fish, skinless chicken and turkey, beans, nuts), you're good.

Fats: you should never eat more than 4 grams of saturated fat per hour of eating. And you should look for products with zero trans fats. Foods containing "partially hydrogenated" ingredients contain trans fats, even if the Nutrition Facts label states "0 grams" trans fat; companies are required only to label trans fats at or above 0.5 grams per serving, so look out for sneaky labeling.

Sodium: unless you have high blood pressure or heart failure, you don't need to worry much about sodium. If you do have high BP, make sure your daily intake is under 1,500 milligrams.

Cholesterol: dietary cholesterol virtually has nothing to do with the cholesterol levels in your blood. You do not need to worry about this number, even if you have high cholesterol (you should be concerned with saturated and trans fats, and syrups and added sugars).

All natural: sugar is natural. So are cyanide and arsenic. That doesn't mean they're good for you. Ignore the phrasing and look at the ingredients.

Whole grain: just because the label says a food "contains whole grains" doesn't mean they're of the 100 percent variety. In fact, companies are allowed to label a product "whole grain" as long as merely 51 percent of it is comprised of whole grains by weight. If you don't see "100%" along with "whole wheat" or "whole grains," the product may have too many simple carbs—which turn to sugar too quickly.

#5 | Find Your Weakness, Create a Substitute

The question that people ask most often of those who have found the way to eat right is "How in the world do you resist [whatever your favorite demon food is]?" That's the sticking point for many people; they just can't imagine their lives without fast-food burgers or large plates of French fries or desserts that have five digits worth of calories. And I'll admit, it's not an easy answer. I have my weaknesses, too. I really, really love chocolate. Put me in the presence of a chocolate molten cake, and I just might melt like a popsicle on a summer day. Every once in a while, if I see fries, I'll think, "Wow, they look awfully good." I've learned to deal with the temptation. For example, I make sure that my chocolate comes in the form of real cocoa, so I don't get the saturated fat from milk chocolate. And if I crave the salty taste of fries, well, then I know I can turn to roasted asparagus. It tastes the same—try a fry or two and roasted asparagus in a blind taste test, and you'll think you had fries. To make the asparagus, cut into two-inch long spears, bathe them in a little rosemary and extra virgin olive oil, put them on a roasting pan in a preheated oven at 275 degrees for twenty-five minutes (you'll have to adjust for your oven), turn and roast for twenty more minutes, and enjoy. By the way, it's not the potato that's bad for you in the fries; it's the oil that they're fried in. Maybe if we could get fast-food chains and restaurants to fry their potatoes in omega-7 oils (with peanut or some other unsaturated oil that withstands the heat of frying), then these fried options wouldn't be quite as hurtful to your body as they are today.

The point here is that to get past these rough spots, you have to identify your weaknesses and then figure out a way to sub in healthy foods that can still satisfy your cravings and taste buds without the damage and destruction that comes from the food felons. To really do the Do-Over, you need to be able to get those unhealthy foods—the ones that can age you and give you wrinkles and impotence—out of your system. That's not necessarily because they are high in calories but because of what these felons do to your proteins and to your genes and to the other chemical processes in your body.

Now, it is worth noting that my biggest food weaknesses weren't chocolate and fries. Nope. Mine came in the form of diet sodas, specifically Diet Dr Pepper. That weakness was so bad that I used to have seven four-foot-by-three-foot pallets (ninety-six cans per palette) of Diet Dr Pepper delivered to my home, because it was cheaper to buy in bulk. That's 672 cans. I would drink one or two on the way to work, many at work, one or two after I played squash, and then several more at night—sometimes hitting thirty to thirty-six twelve-ouncers a day. Crazy. I had a bad habit; some would say I was addicted, but as you'll see in the next chapter, it was really a bad habit. Yes, a very bad habit, but I also guzzled the stuff so that I wouldn't fall prey to my sweet cravings. I did not know then that artificial sweetener may be just as harmful as sugar, though it acts differently in the body. If I needed something sweet, I'd just turn to Diet Dr Pepper. The other advantage was that I drank so much that I could get a lot of steps toward my 10K a day simply from all the trips to the bathroom!

Gradually I slowed down my intake—mostly because I couldn't find a distributor in Cleveland who would deliver it cheaply in bulk when I moved there. I *knew* that more and more research was showing that diet drinks weren't, shall we say, the healthiest of options; the data are mixed, but the common sugar substitutes seem to change the bacteria in your gut to cause insulin resistance. Still, I didn't do anything about it until Mehmet and his wife, Lisa Oz, gave me lots of grief, reminding me that I didn't need to drink it, that it wasn't good for me, that I should give it up. Then, on September 3, 2010, Mehmet and my assistant Beth conspired to put a camera in my office, and Dr. Oz Skyped into my office live for his show and asked me to quit drinking diet soda. I've never had another one.

The reason that I was able to give up my forty-six-year habit was not only because of my buddies checking in on me but also because I was about to find a substitute that could serve a similar role. Immediately, I began drinking coffee. Except for a small percentage of folks who get headaches, abnormal heartbeats, anxiety, or gastric upset from coffee (they are the 12 percent of Americans genetically typed as slow metabolizers of caffeine), the research shows that coffee makes you younger, in that it decreases the chance you'll develop the following age-related diseases: eight cancers, diabetes, Parkinson's, and Alzheimer's. If you're jonesing for java, make sure that it's brewed through a filter; if you don't, it can increase your lousy form of cholesterol. And you can't turn your coffee into a dessert drink with syrups, creams, and other sweeteners, though some natural sweeteners are fine, such as Leaf Stevia and low-fat dairy alternatives like almond milk.

Ideally, though, you'll transition to pure youth-giving black coffee. Almost all genetically fast metabolizers of caffeine get younger from it. It worked for me, because it helped replace the Diet Dr Pepper but still gave my mouth and hands something to do, *and* I liked the taste. I haven't missed Diet Dr Pepper in the four-plus years that I've been away from it. My point isn't that you have to drink coffee. It's that for every vice, addiction, or unhealthy habit, there's a healthy substitution that can meet your needs—and get you on track to make sure your Do-Over is a success.

I certainly can't prescribe a must-do list for every food addiction or preference, but I can give you some guidelines for how to beat it. I like to think of it like this: if you just try to eliminate a certain food, your chances of turning to that food, especially in times of overwhelming stress or emotion, are high. But if you can substitute that aging, energy-robbing food with a good make-you-younger-and-give-you-more-energy food, you'll be much less likely to eat the bad one, because you will have created a new habit, a new taste, and a new response to your stressors or triggers. Some substitution suggestions:

If You Like This . . .	Do-Over with This . . .
Soda	Black coffee or unsweetened green tea
Chips	Crunchy vegetables with sea salt and guac for dipping
French fries	Baked potato skins with olive oil and garlic; roasted asparagus
Pizza	Do-it-yourself (DIY) pizza with 100 percent whole grain crust, marinara, and topped with lots of veggies
Burgers	Salmon burgers or veggie burgers jazzed up with your favorite spices or with grilled onions and peppers
Desserts	Berries mixed with non-fat, no-sugar-added Greek yogurt with a few chunks or sprinkles of dark chocolate

A few more notes about substitutions:

◆ *You Can Retrain Your Taste Buds.* It takes only about two weeks for your taste buds to learn to like a new food. So, if you are committed to your Do-Over, it does take some willingness to experiment with foods you may not be woo-hoo! overjoyed with at first; but with some time (and some nice spices), your new foods can absolutely turn into the ones you love. It happened with me. I didn't used to like salmon, and it's now one of my favorite dishes. I also used to hate spinach, but now that I cook fresh spinach in olive oil and garlic, I love it. People who have switched from whole milk to skim milk know this: they go from whole, to half whole and half 2 percent, to 2 percent, and then to 1 percent, and then to 1 percent with some skim, and then exclusively to skim. By then, they can't imagine drinking whole milk again—just as before, they could never imagine drinking skim. They learned to retrain their taste buds.

- ◆ **You Can Do It When You Eat Out.** Eating out in restaurants is certainly one of the biggest danger zones we have in the quest to do your Do-Over. That's because, to make a grand generalization, they have no vested interest in your health; they have only a vested interest in running their business with foods that can give you immediate pleasure cheaply, but at your long-term expense. But I have found that restaurant owners are willing to work with you on your health needs if you talk to them—and establish a relationship with them. (Remember, you're the CEO!) What I mean is that instead of trying a new place all the time, pick your three or four favorite restaurants and develop relationships with the chefs so that when you come in, they know how you like your food cooked and with what ingredients. They'll adjust to make dishes with olive oil instead of butter, to bring out platters of veggies instead of baskets of bread, to add certain spices to replace sugar. These requests, of course, require educating yourself to know what you want to sub out and what you want to sub in—but you have that knowledge now from earlier in this chapter.

◆ *Experiment with Herbs and Spices.* The reason that we're drawn to fat and sugar is that they give food a lot of flavor and because they're addictive. There's no denying that, and that's one of the biggest challenges we face when dealing with our five food felons. If you try to beat the felon simply by eating lettuce leaves and lettuce leaves alone, you're asking for a midnight gorge on a pound of Pringles. So part of the trick of making flavorful foods is to find great tasting herbs and spices. You can do it for anything. Cinnamon and nutmeg for sweets. Garlic, rosemary, coriander, and turmeric for chicken, fish, and vegetables. Fresh or dried cilantro for bean burritos. The possibilities are endless. But you have to be willing to experiment with new recipes. Have those tasting parties and learn which friends have tastes like yours. Satisfying your taste buds in this way helps extinguish the demons that are tempting you. Even salt is a great choice. Except for the mere 0.33 percent of Americans who have salt-sensitive hypertension, there's nothing to worry about. If your blood pressure is about the ideal (115/75), with or without medications, and stays there when you have some salt, then you're safe to add a little salt to your foods (people with salt-sensitive high blood pressure have major changes in their blood pressure with salt).

◆ **Prepare for an Emergency.** Part of your dietary downfall happens when you open the pints of pudding in times of stress, fatigue, or emotional tumult. And sometimes you can get into trouble simply because you're so hungry that your stomach sounds like a big-cat sanctuary. We all need that backup plan to deal with these emergencies: to know what to grab when your instinct, based on years of bad habits, steers you toward something sugary or saturated fatty. Obviously, you'll have to pick your own in-case-of-emergency list based on what you like, but ideally, these foods should have some crunch and substance to take the edge off.

I have a three-pronged plan: first, I cut up an apple and sprinkle the wedges with a little lemon juice. If that doesn't help, I go to a handful of toasted walnuts that I have pre-prepared to be available to me anytime. Finally, if I'm still famished, I just go through stalks and stalks of celery, perhaps with a little peanut butter or dipped into a bowl of mashed-up garlic. Choose options that are good for you, get you through rough patches, and help you turn the corner in your Do-Over.

◆ **In Extreme Cases, Consider the Alternatives.** I do think that the above tactics will help most figure out ways to substitute healthy foods for disease-promoting ones. However, some people are so badly addicted to foods that these strategies still don't work. One option that I've seen succeed: hypnosis. A man I worked with was so addicted to Cinnabons and macaroni and cheese that he had himself hypnotized to believe that both of those foods were disgusting. (His hypnotist equated them with cat litter.) Now he won't touch them and uses celery as his stress food (oddly enough, he doesn't like cat litter)—he visualizes cat litter each time he sees his past temptations. Another person loved soda so much that he was hypnotized to believe that soda was dog diarrhea. (Sorry!) Unsurprisingly, he can't touch a soda anymore, and now drinks water and coffee.

#6 | Bring In Reinforcements When Necessary

In an ideal world, you'd get all of the nutrition you need from the well-balanced meals you eat; all the vitamins, minerals, and nutrients to power your body every day throughout your life. Unfortunately, most of us are woefully undernourished when it comes to the good stuff and overnourished when it comes to the bad—although I shouldn't even use the word *nourished* when talking about foods that cause impotence or wrinkles or just zap your energy and age you. In fact, 93 percent of people in large surveys in North America do not even get 80 percent of the recommended dietary allowance (RDA) of nutrients, as advocated by the US Food and Drug Administration (FDA) and the US Department of Agriculture (USDA), while 99.9 percent do not get 100 percent of the RDA. That's the main reason to consider taking dietary supplements: to help boost levels in areas where we might be deficient. Now, I serve on the scientific advisory boards of two supplement companies, so I may be biased. Food, of course, is the way we'd like to make sure you get nutrients—often there is a balance of nutrients in food, like magnesium with calcium (see below). But while you're doing your Do-Over (the rest of your life I hope), and if you can't get all the nutrients from food for some reason, I do recommend considering supplements to bridge the gap.

These are the supplements I take and believe should be routine for most men over thirty-five and women over forty-five, because they have either low risk or no risk, or the benefits are greater than the risk.

Vitamin D₃. Between 60 percent and 93 percent of Americans fall short in vitamin D levels, with a level of under 30 nanograms per milliliter of blood. We do know that levels of 35 ng/ml protect against cancer, help reverse diabetes, protect against erectile dysfunction, and help safeguard your arteries from the effects of aging. The most natural source of vitamin D is sunlight, but because of geography and the increased use of sunscreens and sunblocks (a good thing, by the way), most of us don't get the levels we should. I recommend asking your doctor to order a blood test for vitamin D annually, and if you're deficient, find out what dosage of vitamin D supplements you'd need to reach a blood level of 40 ng/ml to 80 ng/ml. Till then, I'd start with 1,000 IU (international units) a day. Toxicity doesn't appear to occur till you reach a level over 110 ng/ml.

Multivitamin. If you have a great diet, you may not need a multivitamin. But the truth is that most of us simply do not get enough from our foods. In addition to vitamin D, many of us are deficient in vitamin E, followed by deficiencies in the mineral magnesium. You can buy a thousand multivitamins for $10, which basically means you need to spend only $3 a year. Since our bodies eliminate excess vitamins and minerals in the urine after twelve hours, it's best to split the dosage into twice a day: half in the morning and half at night. Most men and women over fifty should not take a multi that contains iron because of risks associated with extra iron. In men over seventy, multivitamin use decreases their cancer risk by 18 percent for forms of the disease other than prostate cancer.

Calcium Citrate. The calcium will help in a number of areas, including building bone strength. Since most of us get about half our calcium from food, we need only another 600 milligrams in supplement form to reach the daily recommended amount of 1,200 milligrams. Go too high, and you risk increasing the risk of prostate cancer and probably breast cancer. (Magnesium [300 or 400 mg] is commonly deficient in foods and our blood levels are low, so should be taken with any calcium supplement. Magnesium does decrease the constipation and bloating associated with calcium supplements.)

DHA Omega-3. This nervous system active component of omega-3 helps with brain function and is one of only five things that have been shown to protect your eyes against the first stage of macular degeneration (the others being the nutrients lutein and zeaxanthin found primarily in green, leafy vegetables; avoiding secondhand smoke; and wearing sunglasses outdoors). It converts readily to eicosapentaenoic (EPA) and alpha-linolenic acid (ALA), other forms of omega-3 fats, if your body needs these. I recommend 900 milligrams a day.

Two Baby Aspirin (162 Milligrams Total). Aspirin protects against nine different cancers, including breast, as well as cardiovascular-related conditions such as stroke, heart attack, impotence, and deep vein thrombosis (a condition in which blood clots form, and which can be induced through long airplane flights). The benefits exceed the risks for the typical man over thirty-five and woman over forty-five, but since there are risks, check with your doc beforehand. Take the tablets with a half glass of warm water before and after swallowing to help prevent any gastric discomfort and gastric bleeding that aspirin can cause. And to protect against the same thing happening in your intestine, use one that is not enterically coated. Though there is a theoretic benefit from taking these two babies at night as opposed to in the morning, the best time to take them is anytime you will consistently remember to do so, as there is a rebound effect that increases clotting if you forget them for two days in a row.

Omega-7s. These seem to decrease inflammation and insulin resistance. Interesting note: omega-7s come from macadamia nuts, but it would be way too expensive to produce those oils in pill form from those nuts. But 7s are also found in anchovies; researchers discovered this when they tried to purify the omega-3s from fish oil and found omega-7s in the discarded substances. I recommend 420 milligrams of purified omega-7 a day if you do not enjoy anchovies.

Probiotics. You may know of probiotics as the good-for-you bacteria found in cultured yogurts. We don't have enough data yet to say exactly which type of probiotic you should take as a supplement, but we do know that the variety in bacteria in your gut are crucial to helping metabolize substances you digest for their youth- and energy-giving benefits. We also know that if you have more than four ounces of red meat or six ounces of pork a week or one egg yolk a week, you change the bacterial makeup in your gut to produce chemicals that contribute to arterial aging—more so than elevated blood pressure or lousy LDL cholesterol—and that increases the risks of suffering heart attacks and strokes. Taking a probiotic helps repopulate the bacteria in your gut with the good kind, the kind that can squash some of the bad bacteria's effects. I recommend 4 billion colony-forming units a day.

Coenzyme Q10. This in-cell antioxidant may decrease side effects of the statin drugs that many Americans take to lower their LDL cholesterol and may be beneficial in other ways as well, including reducing diabetes risk and hypertension. It seems to work by helping restore some of the processes involving your mitochondria—the energy centers of the body—though it's not clear exactly how. Perhaps CoQ10 does so by handcuffing molecules called free radicals, which can inhibit mitochondrial function. I recommend 200 milligrams a day.

Note: for women who are potentially pregnant, a prenatal multivitamin is also recommended (half in the morning and half at night, because you urinate out water-soluble multivitamins in fewer than twenty-four hours and you want to keep a stable level throughout the day). Since taking a prenatal three months prior to and during pregnancy is associated with 80 percent fewer congenital abnormalities, 65 percent fewer childhood cancers in offspring of mothers who do so, and 40 percent less autism and autism spectral disorders, this seems like a no-brainer for all women in the potentially pregnant age ranges of twelve to forty-five (50 percent of pregnancies are unplanned in North America). They also seem to improve IQ in the child and decrease depression in moms (since they contain DHA). For men aged eighteen to thirty-five, it isn't clear if there is a benefit from these supplements; it would seem that supplements of calcium, magnesium, and vitamin D are important in building bone strength for all under age thirty-five, and the vast majority do not get adequate amounts in their food choices.

#7 | Buy a Good Freaking Knife— and Learn How to Use It

My job as a wellness coach is not unlike that of track-and-field star Lolo Jones. It's all about getting over hurdles. See, the number one challenge for people trying to do their Do-Over has nothing to do with desire. It has to do with the fear, inconvenience, or struggle to get over whatever hurdle stands in their way. What is the obstacle that's holding you back from changing bad behaviors to good ones?

I've found that the highest hurdle for many people when it comes to eating well is cooking healthy, delicious meals at home. Too much time, too much energy, too much effort. While it could be easy for me to sit here and say, "Get over it, it's worth the investment," the more practical advice is to find the solution that gets you over the hurdle. And what I've found after working with thousands of people is that if you invest in a high-quality knife and learn how to use it quickly and efficiently, your time savings in meal preparation is enormous—and your desire and willingness to make delicious meals increases exponentially.

How so? The key to eating for a Do-Over comes down to integrating more vegetables and fruits into your meals, and the only way you can do that is by cutting them up. (Few of us really eat a pepper like an apple.) So by learning to chop-chop-chop and cut-cut-cut, you give yourself flexibility and variety to prepare delicious foods fast. And the truth is that many people—especially those under forty-five who grew up in the era of prepackaged and overly processed foods—do not know how to hold, let alone use, a good knife. Ask that generation what a Taco Bell spork is, though, and they sure know that! (It's a combined fork and spoon in one utensil if you didn't know.)

I know, I know: you're saying, "Really? One stinking knife will help me avoid buckets of cookie dough, and thousands of dollars in hospital copays and Botox and erectile dysfunction meds?" Well, yes. Of course, eating healthy and avoiding temptation is more nuanced than that, but the knife goes a long way in establishing that environment of wanting to experiment and prepare good foods. I'm willing to bet that if you can cut your prep time in half without sacrificing flavor, then you're just as willing to eat good foods as you are plastic-wrapped nasty ones—especially knowing that you're taking control of your Do-Over.

Here are the essentials of finding and using a good knife:

◆ Size: eight- to ten-inch chef's knife
◆ Approximate cost: $15 to $30
◆ Additions: large cutting boards to give you surface area to cut a lot of vegetables
◆ Cutting technique:

1 Always keep the pointed edge on the cutting board; just lever from the point and cut sliding away from you under the back end.
2 Always cut away from yourself.
3 As you're lining up foods with your noncutting hand, tuck the tops of your fingers under the

bottoms, so you let your knuckles, not your whole fingers, be the guide.

4 See www.realage.com for more cutting instructions, or watch the technique on *YOU: On a Diet*, the PBS special.

Okay, okay, you're thinking that this strategy—buying a good knife—feels simple and silly? Consider Jennifer. She and her husband took up the principles outlined here, and within forty days, she lost about ten pounds, and her husband lost thirty (which is a bit too quickly, actually, because rapid weight loss puts you at a higher risk for gaining it back). She also experienced fewer flare-ups of her osteoarthritis, had more energy, got clearer skin, and looked a whole lot leaner. Plus, she told me, "I also have almost no back fat—you know, that stuff that hangs around your bra!" The key to embracing the diet, she said, was learning how to use a good knife, so that she and her entire family could prepare a salad and veggies for dinner quickly.

It's not just about the knife, it's about what gets you healthy food—fast.

That, I'm telling you, is what will get you a healthy body even faster.

High and Mighty

7 Things You Need to Know
About Detoxifying Your Body

One of the reasons I believe that so many of us don't know how the human body works internally is because it's something you don't ever see up close. It's not as if you can just gaze down and admire the beauty of your intestines, or take a selfie of your carotid arteries in your neck, or open up the hood to take a gander at your brain and see why in the world those dang neurons can't tell you where you left the keys.

It's simply harder to understand what we don't see. Even with textbooks, YouTube videos, and Halloween skeletons to teach us about the body, I know that anatomy and biology can be difficult to grasp (one of the reasons why I included the mini medical school at the beginning of this book). I do think it helps to comprehend biology and the workings of the body by comparing them to things that we do know and can relate to. In that imagery, we can get an understanding of the machinations of the human body so that we can better understand how lifestyle choices can help it or hurt it.

When it comes to thinking about addictions—those repeated actions that we do despite their adverse health effects—I like to explain their effects on the body a little like Jim Cantore might: with the weather. Now, rain in small doses might be good (it helps clean things, helps things grow, and so on), but a monsoon can create a torrent of problems and destruction. We have theories about what starts and propagates an addiction, but these are not definitively proven yet. What we do know is that the toxicity of the substance causes big-time, hurricane-force damage.

In this chapter, I will outline the characteristics of addictions, how they're toxic to our health, and how you can break them; but first, it's important to understand what makes them so destructive. So let's take a look at two of the things we're most addicted to in this country: alcohol and cigarettes. There are many other kinds of addictions that screw with our health, from tanning to cheese fries, but for the sake of this example, I'll use booze and butts. Food addiction, of course, is also rampant; see chapter 3 for details on dealing with nutrition.

We all know the effects of being addicted to cigarettes: you raise your risk of cancer, heart problems, and all kinds of arterial damage that brings about wrinkles, erectile dysfunction, and memory loss, among other things. And with alcohol, you can destroy your liver, as that organ attempts to detox your beverage, as well as harm your heart. The common biological thread in all of these addictions is that they exert a toxic effect in our bodies, by changing our cellular structures and creating inflammation. (And you remember from your mini medical school course that chronic inflammation basically compromises your immune system, causing it to damage your cellular and vascular structures and manifest itself as a host of symptoms and diseases.)

Now, you may want to blame an addiction on your genes—to rationalize that you have no choice but to be addicted to whatever substance it is. While it's true that many of the approximately 20 percent of American adults addicted to alcohol have a genetic disposition to such an addiction, that doesn't mean you can't beat it and have a Do-Over.

But it's not the one cigarette or the one drink. It's the repeated use.

So going back to our weather example, think about the difference between a thunderstorm and a hurricane. With a thunderstorm comes some risk (such as lightning strikes), but there's relatively low risk to the environment or people when a storm comes along. Yes, it can be harmful, but the risks for real damage are relatively low. Same holds true for alcohol and cigarettes. One drink or one cigarette does not provide a knockout punch. In the body, that one cigarette is viewed as a thunderstorm—not ideal, somewhat unpleasant, and it can cause some damage, but it most likely won't cause any long-term problems. Now let's take a look at a slow-moving hurricane that approaches the coastline—and just batters it for hours and hours on end. Power lines come down, houses are destroyed, roads flood and buckle under the pressure, the coastline disappears as the monstrous waves take the sand out to sea. It's systematic destruction on many levels.

That's what an addiction is: It's the constant battering of

powerful forces that destroy the foundation on which your body is built.

If you have to look at our biggest health threats—as a population and as individuals—it truly comes down to these destructive storms in the form of addictions: Addicted to alcohol. Addicted to cigarettes. Addicted to sugar. Addicted to behaviors that induce stress. Addicted to our machines that cause us to skimp on sleep. If you have one of those addictions (or, worse, several of them at once), it's as if your body is simply in the path of a hurricane 24/7—there's no blue-sky relief that comes the day after the hurricane passes. Your body gets battered and battered and battered. Debris flies everywhere, you're flooded with toxins, and your energy systems are shut down. If the addiction continues, the storm never ends.

That said, you absolutely have the power to be the Red Cross, the National Guard, and the politicians with the purse strings: you can provide relief, you can heal the wounds, you can invest in the resources that will rebuild your body—back to your prestorm ideal, as if a storm had never passed through it.

Contrary to what people assume about addictions, you don't have to be stuck with the damage. You can erase the damage. You can heal. After all, isn't this exactly what this book is about: your Do-Over? Nowhere is this more evident than right here. No matter what kind of beating you've put on your body with addictions, you can save it.

Now, I don't want to imply this is easy. I know it's not. And there is a difference between habit and addiction, which

I'll explain shortly. In fact, addiction is truly like a cat-5 hurricane with its sheer force. Strong and scary. Even with my long-term habit of drinking Diet Dr Pepper (or Diet Coke, if I couldn't find a Diet Dr Pepper), I haven't experienced what it feels like to be in the clutches of an addiction, though I've seen plenty of examples up close. (In one of the odder circumstances of my medical career, I knew a colonoscopy doctor who used his endoscope to fish his way through a cabinet with locked drawers to get access to the drugs he was addicted to. He did it so deftly that there was no evidence of a break-in. And even when it was finally found out and he was confronted, he denied that he was stealing drugs. He claimed to be simply practicing his colonoscopy techniques around tight corners, highlighting a classic characteristic of addiction: denial.)

In my job at the Cleveland Clinic—and, really, throughout my entire career—this has been my focus: helping people quiet the storm. In my Breathe-Free stop-smoking program, I have worked with about 2,600 people, and the success rate for those who have stayed smoke-free at the seven-month mark is almost 65 percent. I've also worked with thousands of people to help them break their dietary addictions.

Through this work and the research that has been done on addictive behavior, I know that there's a way to successfully win this biological battle. It does take some time, and it's not as easy as the term "cold turkey" might imply. As is the case with almost anything that helps you turn an unhealthy behavior into a healthy one, it involves a little bit of brain chemistry.

#1 | Understand the Difference Between Addiction and Habit

It may sound like I'm splitting hairs or trying to be a semantics scholar when asking you whether you know the difference between addiction and habit, but I assure you that understanding how and why they're not the same thing is the first step to figuring out your Do-Over.

So why don't we start by playing a little game. I'm going to give you five scenarios, and you get to identify whether they're addictions or not based on the info I've given you (no, you're not allowed more info).

Case 1: Alex drinks more than thirty-two ounces of coffee a day because he likes the taste. He'll drink a large cup in the morning, a large cup in the afternoon, and then a small cup of decaf at night so that it doesn't affect his sleep.

Case 2: Jennifer has at least four alcoholic drinks a day. Last year she started adding vodka to her orange juice in the morning. She blacks out from drinking once a month, and she has missed work several times because of her drinking.

Case 3: Roger takes puffs of a decongestant nasal spray to help unclog his stuffy nose. He started doing it once or twice but has found himself gradually increasing the number of puffs he needs to unstuff his nose.

Case 4: Rachel bites her nails. All. The. Time. At work, at home, in the car, when she's on the phone. She says it helps relieve her stress.

Case 5: Robert and Samantha have been happily married for three years, and they have sex three times a day five days a week.

Okay, take a minute and choose which cases you would classify as an addiction. My guess is that some of you would say that all of them would be classified as addictions. If you did, I would tell you that you were wrong.

For something to be classified as an addiction—and this isn't just clinical speak, this is important in helping you break your destructive behaviors—none of the factors has to do with the volume or amount. It's not the quantity of drinks, for example; it's really about other factors. When we talk about addiction circuitry, it comes down to these factors:

◆ If the behavior has a beneficial effect in the short term but adverse consequences in the long term.

◆ If the person develops a tolerance to the amount of the behavior and then needs more and more of that particular substance or action to achieve those beneficial effects. Let's say you have one or two drinks, start to feel woozy, and always stop there. If you never really increase the volume of alcohol because your body has signaled you to stop, and you never do ongoing or permanent harm to your body, you don't really have an addiction. But if your tolerance rises—you start to need three or four before your body tells you to stop, and then five or six, and then eight or ten, and then you drink all day— that's when those harmful consequences come into play. When tolerance rises and adverse effects occur, it becomes an addiction.

◆ If the person experiences symptoms of withdrawal (the shakes, sweating, extreme anxiety) when he or she tries to stop doing the behavior, this is a sign of addiction.

Now let's look at our five examples through that filter and reevaluate the cases. Which ones are addictions and which ones would now be classified as habits? In the case of our coffee drinker, he certainly drinks a lot of coffee, but the missing piece is adverse effects. There's no health risk to drinking that much coffee, and from what you've read, Alex is not experiencing any jitters or heartbeat abnormalities associated with caffeine, so he's technically not addicted. (However, he could experience withdrawal symptoms— such as a headache—from caffeine if he missed his coffee for a day.) If there is no long-term negative impact, he has no reason to stop drinking that coffee if he likes that coffee.

You likely identified that our vodka-in-OJ drinker has an addiction, as Jennifer has experienced adverse effects in the form of blackouts and missing work. There's no question that her actions would qualify her as an addict. What about Rachel, our nail biter? She does it all the time, so she must be addicted, right? Actually, no. Unless she's a hand model who can't get work or it causes conflict in her relationship, she's not experiencing any adverse effect. So the habit may be excessive, but it's not an addiction. Same holds true for our rabbit-like couple that have sex more times in a week than some couples do in a year. [*Insert applause from the audience.*] To some, that might sound like a full-on sex addiction, but if both partners are happy and like it, there's no addiction—just a fun, healthy habit. Now, if Robert and Samantha weren't on the same mattress—er, page—and one wanted sex three times a day and the other wanted it three times a year, that would undoubtedly cause adverse effects in the relationship, and our morning-noon-and-night person could be straying into addiction territory.

That leaves us with our nasal spray snorter. This one's a bit trickier, but it actually points out very well what addiction is all about. Roger takes the decongestant nasal spray to breathe better, to feel better, to seemingly help his health— so you would assume that's a good action. What's actually happening, though, is that the medication shrinks his mucous membranes to help him breathe easier, but the fallout is that the membranes thicken back up in the absence of the medication. That membrane expansion makes it harder to breathe (this is the effect of withdrawal from the medication), and Roger needs more nasal spray to shrink the membrane again. He's built up a tolerance to that initial puff, and he'll eventually need more and more and more to constantly get that "high" of breathing well.

This example underscores that we could get addicted to anything, really—even if it's inherently good for us. Take exercise. If you work out to the point that you're destroying your joints through overuse and you continue to exercise despite the pain and problems, it might qualify as an addiction.

When it comes down to it, the key part of this process is that our brains search for that high that comes from the immediate pleasure of the act. So when we eat a doughnut and get that temporary surge of dopamine and endorphins, our brains remember: they seek out that flood of pleasure chemicals that make us feel happy. What we don't process is all the shrapnel that hits us afterward, like the lows from plummeting blood sugar levels and the inflammation caused by the added body fat. The trick to breaking the cycle actually comes from the same place: that search for dopamine. The key is trying to find new ways to spur the brain to release dopamine or other chemicals that give us a high but without causing or prolonging addictions.

#2 | To Leverage the Power of Habit to Break the Addiction, You Need to Rewire Your Brain

Many of you, I'm sure, know people who have gone through or are going through very real—and very damaging—addictions. When I think of addictions, one of the first people I think of is a man named Kirk. His family had a long history of alcoholism; his mother died from alcohol-induced liver damage. So Kirk knew he had a family risk. A successful adviser to politicians and business people, he liked writing about wine. He also liked drinking wine and other alcohol. While he didn't experience any adverse effects (he didn't drive when he drank) for a long time, Kirk started developing real signs of alcoholism in his fifties. He'd wake up in the morning, pour himself a Coke, and then put bourbon or scotch in it. Even as he drank throughout the day, he stayed successful and cogent and funny in his job.

But then Kirk blacked out several times and knew he had to get some help. He went into an alcohol-addiction treatment program and successfully stopped drinking alcohol. About three years into his recovery, he relapsed, when an attempt at moderation failed: he started with a glass of wine and by the end of the weekend, Kirk was so blotto that he knew he could never do moderation. Now he's been alcohol free for about five years. In addition to taking anticraving medication and attending a peer support group, Kirk took up walking and exercising, which he credits greatly with having helped him kick his addiction.

The reason breaking addictions poses such a biological test is that repeated and addictive behavior actually changes your brain circuitry: when you learn a behavior, neurons communicate with one another, telling you, "This is how you do the task," whatever it might be. New connections are made to enable you to add numbers, solve problems, translate foreign languages, serve a tennis ball, learn guitar chords—anything.

Two things happen when you're learning that skill or action. One, the connections between those neurons strengthen. Use those neurons, and they become tough so that the once-difficult skill becomes easy. It's why learning piano may be difficult at first, but then you practice and practice until the damn neighbors are so sick of hearing "Chopsticks" that playing the song becomes second nature. Your neurons know what to do and do it quickly. It's an example of biological efficiency: you need energy at first to learn the behavior, but not so much once you know it.

Two, while those connections between neurons are strengthening, the ones you aren't using are being whittled away. It's the whole "Use it or lose it" maxim. Let's say that you learned Spanish in elementary school but haven't used a lick of it since. If you try to remember it when you're fifty-five, you may sputter a few words or phrases, but you won't recall much at all. Those neurons said essentially, "This bozo knows *nada* about Spanish, so why are we wasting our time firing off '*uno, dos, tres, cuatro*' to one another? Forget about it. We're outta here." And in the process, you lose those connections; you lose that ability.

So how does this apply to addictions and habits? When you're addicted to drinking or cigarettes or Lucky Charms, it works the same way. The repeated behavior rewires your brain to perform that action like you do when you learn to play Beethoven's Fifth. I eat, therefore I smoke. I talk on the phone, therefore I smoke. I have sex, therefore I smoke. (Afterward, hopefully.) You have created the brain circuitry to reinforce those unhealthy habits because your brain wants the temporary high that comes from them, no matter the damage that follows.

Therefore, the answer lies in the problem. We need to use

that same circuitry to discover new habits that allow us to build new connections, so that the destructive ones can be pruned. But here's the thing: you can't expect the cigarette or other addictive circuitry to whittle away by itself; you have to put something in its place. You have to find new circuitry boards to build, so that your brain stops investing its energy in the connections that make you want to do the destructive behavior, like smoke. This is where the power of habit comes into play. Remember, habit can be a repeated behavior that gives you a high, as in our coffee-drinker example. As long as there are no adverse effects associated with that repeated habit, then you are going to rewire your brain away from the addiction and into a healthy habit.

Now, I don't especially care what that new habit is, as long as it is not destructive; but better still if it is healthful. For Kirk, it was exercise. For others, it's clicking a pen every time they want a cigarette. And sometimes it's conditioning the brain to want to eat baby carrots every time you're about to dive into a bag of chips. For a lot of people, it's the ten thousand steps a day. So pick whatever habit you like, you want, and that will give you some kind of high—without the adverse effects. This is the way you morph an addiction into a healthy habit.

You're not trying to outmuscle your brain chemicals by resisting the very real and very powerful urges that come from our addictive substances. But you are trying to out-smart them.

#3 | Cold Turkey Often/ Usually Doesn't Work

If you want to know how trying to quit an addiction cold turkey usually works out, consider this story: a CEO of a company, a heavy drinker, did most of his drinking about four blocks from his home, so that he could navigate his way home in his SUV. Figuring that those four blocks were short enough to operate on autopilot, he never thought he'd have a problem, even after drinking too much.

Well, one day he finally realized that he had a drinking problem and decided to quit cold turkey. Didn't tell anyone. Didn't ask for help. Didn't follow any formal program. He decided to go solo. Two days later, he woke up in a crashed SUV surrounded by police cars. It turns out he didn't re-member a thing: that he had relapsed after two days and went to his usual spot at the bar, that he paid the bill and got into his SUV, but this time he got on and off the freeway to his office and had weaved through traffic. Someone alerted the police about his erratic driving, and, in fact, he ended up smacking his car into something. (He doesn't remember do-ing that but had done $15,000 worth of damage to his SUV.) He ended up spending the night in jail for drunk driving, and his family reached out to me to help with an interven-tion, so this story—as I write this—is a work in progress. Luckily, nobody was hurt, and things could have been much worse for him—and many other innocent people.

I tell you this story not to scare you or wag my finger in disapproval, but to reinforce the fact that this is the type of tale I hear all the time when people try to quit cold turkey. When our brains search for that addictive substance, it simply relapses to what it knows: the addiction. Cold turkey is as effective as a campfire in a rainstorm. It just doesn't work.

Now, there are some outlier cases where quitting cold turkey succeeds because the addicted person makes it his or her mission to stop, and does have the willpower to overcome the brain circuitry. However, the fact is that most people who successfully break the chains of addictions over the long term (*long term* being the key word) can't just stop abruptly—because of the wiring system that I explained in the last section. Your body and brain need time to drop the learned connections and build new ones. Not only is going cold turkey misunderstood, but it's also misused. None of my addiction-breaking programs involves cold turkey. A couple of things have to be in place in order for the addiction to be broken—namely, that a new habit has to be started, as well as perhaps some chemical help. That's why many antiaddiction programs include some kind of anticraving prescription drug, such as bupropion or a benzodiazepine. When you take those drugs, it helps mitigate the withdrawal symptoms that you feel when trying to come off an addiction, giving your brain time to break down those entrenched wires so that you can rewire your brain with healthy habits.

It should be noted that different drugs are used for different addictions, because they're designed to work on the mechanism that causes addiction. For example, bupropion (we recommend in a lower and different dose than in the brand name preparation, Zyban) is used in cigarette cessation programs because it quiets the addictive properties of nicotine. For added sugar addictions, we look not to med-ication, but rather other foods. Your body needs sugar to function; and your brain, eyes, and some sex organs rely on it exclusively for their energy. Therefore, we try to cut out heavy doses of sugar that come from refined carbohydrates. By eating foods that give you a "slow drip" of sorts (such as 100 percent whole grains), your body can then use sugar, but not in the shotgun approach that comes from simple sugars and added syrups. In a way, those healthy whole grains act as medication.

So what's the take-home? To successfully overcome ad-diction, you will likely need to enlist the help of a health care specialist, if for nothing else than to prescribe medica-tion temporarily to help you get past the initial tension and discomfort. Cold turkey may seem like the heroic thing to try. "Yes, I did it all by myself! No help at all! I was able to throw twelve packs of cigarettes down the toilet, never to touch one again!" But you know what? I'm not in the busi-ness of trying to create mythical heroes. I'm in the business of helping you achieve your Do-Over—not by six o'clock tonight but through methods that will last your entire life-time. Remember, going cold turkey doesn't mean a thing if you're back puffing away two weeks later.

You'll see the specifics of my plan in just a few pages, and this will walk you through the 210-day program that will help you get started on that Do-Over. Part of being suc-cessful on that program is acknowledging that cold turkey should be chucked down the garbage disposal.

Just look at the numbers. The data show that people who try to quit smoking cold turkey have only a 2 percent success rate. If you try to kick the habit using just an anticraving pill, there's a 3 percent to 5 percent success rate. If you use an anticraving medication and a nicotine patch, the success rate rises to about 10 percent. But if you use all three, plus substitute another habit to take the place of the addictive behavior (like 10K a day of steps), and enlist the support of a buddy, the success rate soars to over 30 percent. As I mentioned before, the success rate in our study of more than 2,600 tobacco users was an astounding 63.8 percent. Is it perfect? Of course not. But I'll take my chances with a nearly two-in-three success rate over just two success stories per every hundred patients any old day of the week.

#4 | It's Good to Get High

You may have seen enough Cheech and Chong movies to associate getting high with loopy language and a watch-the-world-go-by attitude. Especially when it comes to illegal drugs, for many of us parents, we've spent as much time saying "Don't do drugs" as we've spent asking "Do you want the crusts cut off your PB&J?" For good reason, too. The chemicals that produce highs in illegal drugs (and prescription drugs used illegally, like OxyContin) have been found to increase the risk of many different problems, ranging from mental issues to reduced motor skills (putting people at risk if they drive), as well as leading to addictive patterns that bring about even more problems.

Certainly the use of medical marijuana and its legality in many states have brought more attention to marijuana than ever before. It's my opinion that unless you have medical conditions for which marijuana is prescribed, the risks in habitually using recreational marijuana—certainly for brains that are under twenty-one in women and under twenty-four in men—outweigh the benefits.

Here's the issue: it's not the high that's bad. It's the high we're after.

What we're after is that surge of endorphins or dopamine to make us feel good, feel happy, feel connected with the world. We can get that high from a number of different delivery mechanisms: a brownie, a run, sex, a great piece of music, vodka, a cigarette, a cup of tea, anything.

The dopamine isn't bad. The high isn't bad.

We should be doing things in our life to chase highs.

The thin line exists, however, because of the consequences associated with the mechanisms that deliver those highs. Alcohol may give you a high, but it may impair your cognition so much that you get into a fight or behind the wheel. Cigarettes may give you a high, but they're also happy to turn your lungs into what looks like the site of an oil spill. Doritos may give you a tongue-gasm, but if you eat bag after bag, well, you know how that gut-busting story goes.

I think part of this battle comes down to how you frame the challenge. For some reason, we rationalize that if we have to give up the thing that gives us pleasure, we'll decrease our quality of life. But the reality is that you absolutely shouldn't think of quitting an addiction as giving up your pleasure points. Your mission needs to be finding new ones. After all, it's not the high that's different; it's only the way you get there that needs to change.

#5 | Recovery Is Lifelong

I like delivering bad news about as much as I like the idea of kids gorging on jelly doughnuts. Which is to say, not very much. As I've said, I spend most of my life trying to be as cheerleader-positive as I can. But sometimes, well, we have to tell it straight. And this is that time: recovery isn't something you go on and off. You don't take vacations from recovery. You don't get a free pass to smoke on Saturday and stay smoke-free every other day. You don't get to binge on your addiction if you promise to stay clean right after that. You don't get a reward for being good. But what you do get is your Do-Over. Much more fun and valuable.

You know how some people say they're on a diet and then off a diet? (I hate that, too, by the way.) The successful people know that healthy isn't about following a strict plan for four weeks and then straying into the land of bonbons for a few weeks, only to hunker down for another four weeks and then reward yourself with apple pie after you've lost a few pounds. Same goes for conquering addiction. It's not easy. It's not temporary. And it's not about flipping switches on a whim. If you want to make sure that you rewire your brain permanently, you have to continue to build and cultivate those connections with healthy habits. Because once you fray the wires with the addictions, you risk making your whole system go haywire again.

I do know that replacing addictions with healthy habits is the key component, next to a buddy, for making this work. But I don't want to give you the impression that it's as simple as picking up a bag of broccoli, swapping it for your pack-and-a-half-a-day cigarette habit and saying, "Woo-hoo, we're all good!"

So much of being successful with your Do-Over, I believe, isn't just about what actions you take, but about your mind-set before you take and while you're taking those actions. And one of the key truths that you have to wrap your brain around is this: it's doable, but there aren't shortcuts. Your brain chemistry can work in your favor, so it's not as hard as you think. But you also have to know that you can't slip up. That's where the secret lies. When you retrain your brain, you'll decrease the chances of making mistakes, acting on impulses, and giving your brain a reason to direct you toward that plate of fried and loaded potato skins. You'll have taught your brain how to get high without the damage that comes from some of our more addictive toxins. You do not want your brain rewired from one moment of having succumbed to temptation. That one moment enables more moments when you feel like you've failed. If you do have a slip-up—and many do—forgive yourself fast and get back on the health wagon.

#6 | You *Can* Stop Smoking

The worst smoker I ever saw: a high-profile lawyer in Chicago. He smoked five packs a day. Let me repeat: Five. Packs. A. Day. Basically, the only time he wasn't smoking was when he was asleep or eating—actually putting food into his mouth. He smoked so much that he often double-fisted with a cigarette in each hand. He'd light his new cigarette with the end of his still-smoldering butt.

Since he did a lot of work for the city, which had recently debated and was near a decision to prohibit smoking in its offices, Evan decided to quit. He had called me because he had heard from a friend that I helped people stop smoking. So I put him on the program that I'm including below. I coached him on the phone and via email in later years. And he did it: stopped for good, with the exception of one puff he took in a bar. (He felt so bad about it that he ran out of there and called me immediately!)

About four months after Evan quit, he called me and said, "Mike, I just had the greatest dream. It was the greatest night, and I died and went to heaven, and I got to smoke in heaven. And you don't know how great it was! Those cigarettes were so good."

My response: "First of all, I know what you do, and there's no way you're going to get into heaven. And two, it probably wasn't heaven, because there's no way they have tobacco there." Yes, I joked with him, but my experience with Evan taught me two very important things: one, tobacco addiction is incredibly powerful; so powerful that people can feel this high from the very first puff. If you haven't experienced it yourself, you can underestimate how powerful that pull to smoke is, and so the addiction-breaking program has to be solid to help you avoid a relapse. And two, it taught me that, wow, if Evan can do it—at five packs a day—anyone can do it. Evan gave up his cigarettes, and by my estimates, he lived eighteen years longer than he would have had he continued to smoke. He reversed signs of heart disease and emphysema. He died suddenly around the age of seventy-five from abnormal heart beats while he was gardening in his backyard, but given his smoking habit and destruction, I believe that he had been on pace to die well before he turned sixty. He reversed the damage. He got a Do-Over. And he beat back one of the most powerful addictions out there. I believe that you can, too.

Here's my Breathe-Free program, which has worked for more than 60 percent of the people who have followed it. But you have to realize that it's not an overnight fix. It can take up to six months to feel fully recovered, with the addiction banished successfully from your brain.

Smoking Cessation Plan

1 Get a buddy. (See chapter 1 for how to select your buddy; this is the secret sauce of your Do-Over.)
2 Start walking thirty minutes extra every day, no excuses. *Every day.* Start this on Day 1, one month before quitting.

3 Call or email your buddy every day to confirm that you walked. If you miss two days, restart the day count at Day 1.

4 Ask your doctor for prescriptions for 100-milligram bupropion tablets and also nicotine patches dosed according to the amount you smoke. For a half-pack-a-day habit, it's 7 milligrams to 10 milligrams; for a half pack to one pack, 14 milligrams; for one to two packs, 21 milligrams to 22 milligrams. For more than two packs a day, ask your doctor.

5 On Days 28 and 29, take one bupropion.

6 Day 30: it's your stop-smoking day. Apply your nicotine transdermal patch system: one patch on your arm, chest, or thigh. Replace daily.

7 On Day 30 and all subsequent days, take bupropion each morning and each evening. Most folks wean off bupropion between days 90 and 180.

8 Continue walking thirty minutes extra or more each day and call your buddy. Feel free to drink as much coffee, tea, and/or water as you wish.

9 Phone or email your buddy daily to discuss your overall progress.

10 Begin weight lifting on Day 60 or earlier. Do not increase your physical activities by more than 10 percent per week.

11 Decrease patch size by one-third every two months.

12 After six months, decrease to one bupropion tablet in the evening; when you hit seven months, discontinue the drug completely.

13 Carry one bupropion tablet with you at all times, in case you feel a craving.

#7 | Your Best Prescription: Oxytocin

If you think that the above line is an oxymoron, then you've got the wrong oxy. Oxy*codone*, better known by its trade name, OxyContin, is a highly addictive narcotic painkiller. But oxy*tocin* is the chemical that you *want* to get addicted to. Oxytocin is the feel-good hormone that's released when you bond with others; it's often referred to as the "mothering hormone" because the pituitary gland secretes it when babies and mothers bond.

The reason you want to become addicted to oxytocin is because this is one of the vital elements of dealing with and fighting addiction: drawing on the support, encouragement, and occasional smackdowns from your buddy. I won't spend much more time on this because it's the subject of chapter 1, but it's important enough for me to remind you that it's my experience (and the research supports this) that you will face a far harder time breaking the spell of addiction if you try going it alone. It's one of the reasons that many addiction-recovery programs utilize group settings and group formats for sharing stories of success and failure—because the way to fight really powerful, harmful chemicals is to swap in really powerful helpful ones like oxytocin. That's done through forming relations with other people, and one of the main reasons why your first Do-Over deed is all about making sure you have an ally on your side.

A resident in the department of anesthesiology that I chaired got addicted—along with his girlfriend—to propofol, a drug that helps you relax and is administered prior to and during surgery. It's the same drug that killed Michael Jackson. (Side note: anesthesiologists are at very high risk of drug addiction because of their easy access to these kinds of pain-numbing drugs.) One day a colleague came up to me and told me that we had a problem: there were pools and pools of blood all over the bathroom that the resident doctors use.

"What the hell happened?" I asked. After some deduction and investigation, we figured out that one of the residents must have had an addiction to propofol and injected himself and his girlfriend to receive the drug intravenously while having sex. (It is reported to intensify orgasm.) Something must have gone wrong, like the IV tube coming out during the act, which caused blood to volcano all over the place.

Needless to say, we, as a department, had to stage an intervention with the resident. There were obvious adverse effects involved in this addiction—he would risk losing his medical license for drug abuse—so we called him into my office. You know what he did? Didn't fight. Didn't deny it. Just walked in and said he was ready to pack his bags and get some help. Amazing! That doesn't happen all that often during an intervention. But it also points to a real issue when it comes to addiction: no change is going to happen until the addicted person is out of denial and ready to make a change. Sometimes that change can be prompted by loved ones (more reason why oxytocin is so important), but ultimately, the addict has to be ready to take the first step of many that will free him or her from addiction. In this case, it also helped that the resident was able to convince his girlfriend to join him in therapy.

The kicker: he and the woman beat the addiction. She's in the medical field, and he's now a faculty member at a major university. Best: they're married with a couple of kids and living happily and healthily.

To me, there were a couple of factors that really helped the two of them beat it. They had certainly gotten themselves into a bad and potentially life-destroying situation. But they were able to acknowledge that they needed help, were willing to accept it, and then got help together.

Together is the key word. Be in it together with someone. Doesn't have to be your spouse. Doesn't have to be someone who's at the very same stage as you. Doesn't even have to be the same addiction. But it does have to be someone else who can help you, inspire you, pull you, and push you. That's because addiction is one mountain that's pretty damn impossible to climb solo.

Frazzled? Dazzle!

7 Things You Need to Know About Stress Management

When it comes to health doctrines, we accept many of them as absolutes: broccoli is good, cigarettes are bad, and never ever—under any circumstances—should you perform a knee replacement on yourself. More often than not, we're correct: most of our health mantras come about after years of science have confirmed some variation of a + b = c. But every once in a while, an accepted directive will get flipped on its head, and we'll reverse our thinking—as with coconut oil or coffee. Or maybe we don't have enough data to really know the answer yet, which is true of just about all of our yet-to-be-cured diseases or issues such as how often women should have mammograms. Sometimes, however, health messages that we hear day after day are either wrong, outdated, or just poorly framed.

Stress falls into this category.

For too long, we've been hammered with the message

that stressful events are bad, and therefore you must prevent stress. Right? Stressful events get compared with rough ocean seas, battering your brain, disturbing your life, and churning up all kinds of angst that wreak biological havoc on your body. What you need, the thinking goes, is tranquillity: flat-as-glass water where there's no chop, no disruption. Just a peaceful existence that allows you to sit back and watch the sun rise and the sun set, idling your life away.

Well, I'm calling bull bolus on that message. At least part of it.

While it's absolutely true that stressful events can mix up your innards like a blender (more on that in a moment), the wrongly framed message is that the only way to stop the turmoil is to avoid stress and settle down to an easy-peasy existence. The end goal is not to bubble-bath your way through every day.

Case in point: imagine your life with no stress. Say you picture yourself on a Caribbean island with no electronics, floating away on a raft with a piña colada in one hand and your partner's hand in the other. Sounds wonderful, right? My guess is that you'd get bored—maybe after a week, maybe after a month, maybe after a year. But at some point, you'd go crazy, because you need the challenges of life to keep you stimulated, engaged, and passionate about what you do and who you are. So the point is not to *avoid* stressful events but to minimize the impact of stress on you. You want to absorb the stress like a shock absorber going over a pothole rather than trying to outsmart it like a cat burglar. And when you rethink what stress really is and does—and how you're supposed to handle it—that's what helps change your body and your health so that you can have your Do-Over, so that the evil effects of stress don't mess up your body.

Now, the tricky part when it comes to stress is that, at least at this point, it's not like some of the other areas of biology that we can address. I can tell you that eating *x*, *y*, and *z* foods will help ease inflammation and improve your overall health. And I can tell you that walking ten thousand steps a day will also reverse some of the destructive processes that are going on in your body. But stress isn't like curing appendicitis. No single prescription works for everybody. And unfortunately, there's no 400-milligram dose of Thai massage that will automatically help all people manage their stressors better. So what do you do? This, admittedly, is sort of like experimental medicine—except in this case, you're the doc, and you have to figure out what prescription works best for you.

#1 | Your Body Knows How to Handle Stress

There are days, no doubt, when you feel like your head is going to explode. All the bits of information that you're trying to absorb feel as if they're bubbling so raucously that they're seeping out of your nostrils and oozing out of your ears until finally you just can't take it anymore, and: *ka-blam-o!* We all know that feeling. We all experience inordinate amounts of stress, no matter our age, gender, and social status. Although we can categorize stress into some broad categories (more on that in a moment), it comes in many forms particular to our own lives.

We all *get* what stress feels like. But here's something that most of us don't realize: your body, at least evolutionarily, knows exactly how to handle stress, even if *you* don't have the slightest clue.

What do I mean by that? Well, when the body is under stress, it reacts by helping us get out of the situation. In generic terms, this is the fight-or-flight response. In biological terms, it's actually quite masterful.

As noted in mini medical school, a few thousand years back in time, when you could find yourself locking eyes with a sharp-toothed beast, you had two choices if you didn't want to end up as a Paleolithic appetizer: you get the heck out of there, or you say, "Let's go, big boy, want some of this?" You flee or you face off. Here's the thing: Your body can do neither in its normal, everyday, ho-hum state. How the heck are you supposed to summon the capacity to bolt out of a dangerous situation or punch with hammer-like power if you're peacefully lollygagging along in life?

So your body essentially pushes the red emergency button to activate your stress response. Your heart rate increases, and your blood pressure increases, and a series of hormonal responses kick in—giving your body the power to run or to strike. The emergency button sends out your biological troops to take care of you (evolutionarily, to insure the reproduction of our species). All of those responses are a good thing; it's what allows blood to pump and energy to get to your muscles to take care of the task in front of you. It raises your energy and alertness, as well as your blood sugar to fuel your muscles and give you the wherewithal to get away. And when you're done and safely back at home, disaster averted, your system quiets down and goes back to its chilling-on-a-rock state of happiness. Your body worked in overdrive to save your butt, and now it's time to relax.

Now fast-forward to a time when sharp-toothed animals come in the form of deadlines, bosses, hectic schedules, in-laws, health issues, divorce, kids getting in trouble at school, and all the zillion other things that can cause you stress. Those problems linger. You can't always fight or flee and be done with the problem in front of you. If you're typical, you grapple with constant problems—and sometimes the answers aren't as easy as belting the beast in the snout and making a run for it. So what happens biologically? The emergency button isn't on for a short period and then off. It's on all the time. And that means your heart rate soars, your blood pressure increases, your hormone levels elevate—for longer periods than they're designed to. That's what causes stress-related health problems. It's not the momentary stress response. It's the chronic stress response.

Take, for example, our wonderful caregiving nurses at the Cleveland Clinic: they work like crazy and care so much about their patients that they often postpone bathroom breaks for hours. But you know what stresses them the most? It's the things they can't control that are chronic: the repeated twenty- to forty-second delays when they have to log onto each new patient's computerized electronic medical record (EMR), or move from from one patient's room to another and have to wait that twenty to forty seconds for their computers to reconnect thirty or more times a day. We're going to have to find a way of fixing that so our nurses don't have to deal with this cause of chronic stress, or at least have a meditation or song or whatever helps them automatically appear on their iPhones every time they have to wait to log in.

Whatever your causes of stress, those elevated heart rates, blood pressure, and hormone levels have a direct effect on your health. Increased cortisol and epinephrine (two of the stress hormones that rise when your pituitary gland tells your adrenal glands that you're under duress, as described in mini med) raise your blood sugar (so your muscles have energy to run or punch). But that increase now messes up the protein that forms the grout-like substance between the tile-like cells in the inner layer of your arteries, making them more vulnerable to high blood pressure and making it more likely they develop tears or nicks. Remember from our mini medical school that once arteries tear or sustain damage, the body tries to repair them by sending lousy LDL cholesterol laden fatty streaks, which become (over years or even decades) plaques and then blockages. That furthers the process of increasing blood pressure and your risk for heart attacks, strokes, wrinkles, impotence, memory loss, and other cardiovascular problems. What about all that blood sugar? Comes in handy when you need to urgently scale a tree to get out of the jawline of an angry alligator. But in a state of chronic stress, that excess blood sugar has to go somewhere, and that somewhere is usually in the form of damaging belly fat, which causes inflammation and impairs your infection-fighting defense system. You also raise your risk of developing diabetes, as well as autoimmune diseases and cancer. What's more, cortisol decreases your memory reserve by pruning your brain connections.

Stress isn't damaging in its own right. And it's not damaging because it makes you depressed and frustrated and anxious, although those reactions are all very destructive in their own right. The greatest harm stems from the domino effect of the chemical reactions caused by chronic stress. So when you joke that all your responsibilities are going to make you have a breakdown, that is literally what's happening: your body is breaking down.

The first thing to learn when thinking about how to get your stress under control is this: In terms of how your body ages and gets damaged, stress shouldn't be defined as the event itself, but rather, your reaction to the event.

The goal here is to mitigate the stress response so that, biologically speaking, your body isn't in an infinite freak-out state.

#2 | Learn from Your Loincloth-Loving Ancestors

You live in stressful times. You know it, and the data support it. Some research measures our collective stress levels on a perceived stress scale—that is, people self-report how stressed they feel. One such scale runs from −10 to +30, and subjects were asked to report how stressed they felt, using that scale (with −10 roughly equaling rocking on a hammock in the Bahamas and +30 roughly equaling your brain feeling like Mount Vesuvius). From 1979 to 1983, fewer than 5 percent of the population reported levels greater than 20. Now? More than 50 percent do. A tenfold increase. Tenfold!

So what, you say? That's just people whining and moaning about how hard they have it. Maybe. Such is the case with self-reported studies; they do have some flaws. But here's the kicker: those with the highest levels of perceived stress developed the most chronic disease.

Perhaps that was because people tried to self-medicate with food, and thus all of those negative effects of overeating kicked in, Or perhaps it was due to all of those chemical stress responses taking place. It's a very real problem, akin to any other so-called major disease or condition. It's just that stress is very difficult for science and doctors to measure in the same hard numbers way that we can measure your blood pressure, blood sugar, T cells, or many other indicators of many health problems.

While there are many possible solutions to help mitigate the stressors in your life (more on that below), I do think there's one underrated solution—a solution that's not very sexy and doesn't involve yoga mats or vanilla-scented bath salts or the strong hands of Masseur Hans.

You want to know what it is?

Solve. The. Problem.

Think about what our caveman brethren did when faced with the stress of that gnarly-looking beast. They dealt with it right then and there—either by getting away or beating it away. They didn't say, "Hang on a second, I'm gonna sit on the rock and watch an episode of *Keeping Up with the Cavedashians*, and we'll deal with your ten-inch claws sometime tomorrow." They didn't prolong the stress. They faced it. Granted, sometimes they lost the fight, but the lesson we can take from them is that the best way to keep your stress levels at bay is not to ignore the problem but to work out a solution. Sometimes it's confronting an uncomfortable issue head-on, sometimes it's delegating a problem to someone else, sometimes it's asking the whole tribe to get in on the fight with you. But you'd do yourself a whole world of good if you would confront your issues instead of ignoring them or procrastinating.

Avoiding issues drains your energy. Deal with the stressor first thing in the morning or schedule it into your day so that it's not hanging over your head. Also, as your day gets busier, it's easier to put off until tomorrow, tomorrow, to-morrow. Deal with it before it tosses you around like a row-boat in a storm. If it's a stressor that you've let linger for too long: maybe months, years, or even decades, consider what it would be like for you to take an action to resolve it. You may feel a certain unease, fear, or outright dread, and that's okay—remember that *you* have the power to take an action, and often our fears are scarier than the actual action we're avoiding. Whether confronting it resolves it or not, if you don't go for it, you can be sure it will keep being the way it has been.

Consider the case of one my patients, Nancy, who owned a sports bar. She was known for her elaborate works of art when it came to creating nachos—as in, they were so popu-lar that people requested all kinds of crazy creations, so she made them in all shapes and forms. But the stress of keep-ing up made her feel crazy, too! She grew more and more stressed trying to keep up with all of the requests—to the point where she couldn't even sleep much anymore because she worried so much about what her next nacho creation would be. Then one day she woke up and decided that was it. No more nachos. *Nada más!* Even though people loved what she did, they were causing her angst, stress, and sleep trouble. Not wanting her health to suffer or her culinary art to degrade, Nancy just decided to eliminate the stressor. Now, maybe there were quite a few patrons unhappy with Nancy's decision, but her health benefited from it. Her troubles simply went away when she eliminated the source of her worry.

There is a big difference between what Nancy did and what some people can do when it comes to stress: she had control. As the bar owner, she had the authority to throw up her hands, wash the cheese off of them, and say she's not going to do it anymore. Research shows clearly that the more autonomy someone has in his or her job, the lower the risk of heart disease and the lower the risk of other stress-related issues. That's easier said than done, for many folks. It's not like you can just tell your boss that you're in charge now, and you can't just suddenly quit everything and go open a banana boat company in the Caribbean. But if you can hunker down into an aspect of your job over which you have control, you'll likely be better off in the long run. That doesn't mean that jobs with control have zero stress, but it does mean that those who wield the power usually have better health outcomes in the area of stress management.

Now, I don't mean to give short shrift to people's stressors. Not every problem can be floored with a metaphorical right hook, but I can say that even just attempting to solve your stressor is more beneficial to your biology than simply hoping that the problem goes away. So no matter what form of stress relief you enjoy and find helpful for you, nothing beats going back to the biological basics: you quiet your stress response best not when you unplug from the world but when you unplug your stress response from the stressor.

#3 | The Best Stress Response: Whatever!

If I had a prescription pad and could write down the perfect concoction to combat stress, the first order I'd write is what I just said: solve the issue if you can. But after that, my prescription pad would have a whole lot of fill-in-the-blanks—because, really, you're the only one who can decide what the best technique for managing your response to a stressful event will be. Unlike diet, where there are clear-cut good and bad choices, stress relievers can come in different forms. The only question here is that you obviously don't want to choose something that causes harmful health problems, like so many so-called stress relievers such as cigarettes, alcohol, TV, excessive ice cream, TV with excessive ice cream, and other bad-for-your-body vices that can turn into addictions.

But other than those things, anything goes. What you're after are activities that will calm your brain—some by releasing dopamine, one of the feel-good neurotransmitters. Now, dopamine won't actually break up blood sugar or decrease blood pressure. But what it does is decrease your perception of, and subsequent reaction to, stressful events. So something that may have felt like a whack-attack stressor may now seem like only a minor blip once you're in a state of a dopamine high. And if you perceive a stressor to be less daunting, then that's how your body reacts, too: you don't get all the Defcon 5 levels of chemical reactions going on in your body. That's why solving those stress-inducing issues is so important. It's almost like an air bag for your body—it softens the blow.

You name it, anything can get you to release dopamine in that feel-good way: Massages, exercise, walks, baths, yoga, chatting with a friend, meditation, mindful breathing, dancing, sipping tea in a quiet room, petting a dog, guided imagery, scrunching up all of your muscles and then releasing them, having sex with your partner, having sex with yourself, squeezing a stress ball, gardening, hiking, cooking—you get the picture. The trick is to find the activity or activities that calm down your biology. And that's what gets you your Do-Over: freeing your body from the battering of prolonged stress.

To learn how to calm your stress system, you have to learn how it gets activated in the first place. This is the typical cycle:

Part One. An event sets you off. It can be very different things for each of us, so it might be a personal comment that someone made, someone close to you getting sick, a situation that evokes strong emotions that make you feel uncomfortable. Anything. Your hormones kick into action.

Part Two. You respond to the event and those activated hormones with physical symptoms. These can include subconsciously holding your breath, stroking your beard or face, rocking back and forth, indigestion, headache, grinding your teeth (chewing pens for me), itching, neck and shoulder pain, muscle tension, increased pain in your joints (or anywhere else), sweaty palms, increased hot flashes or flushes, nausea, dizziness, racing heart rate, constipation, poor concentration, impaired memory, difficulty sleeping, and insomnia.

Part Three. Your physical symptoms trigger emotional symptoms. You may experience negative thinking, increased self-doubt or insecurity, loss of meaning or purpose, worry, rebellion, or even a screw-you attitude. You may feel like a victim or as if you've lost control, like you are inefficient, stuck in life, edgy, wanting to be a martyr, like you don't belong, depressed, lonely, bored. The story connected to the trigger and the feelings engendered by the physical response and your hormonal responses are amplified. This leads to:

Part Four. You turn to behavioral attempts to self-soothe. Many of these self-soothing behaviors are destructive, such as eating within two and a half hours of a previous meal, smoking, indulging in fatty/sugary/salty foods that sap your energy, shopping, excessive drinking, drunk shopping, gambling, taking drugs, watching mindless TV (however some TV, like *The Dr. Oz Show*, isn't mindless), exercising excessively, overworking yourself, acting controlling or bossy, and being gruff with those you should care about. These changes in the fourth part of the cycle then reinforce events that set you off again, like arguing with someone about eating habits, or passing in front of a mirror, or thinking to yourself that you have less self-worth. Those feelings and events continue the cycle until you learn to self-soothe or manage the stress in a positive way.

Here's how you can break that normal response so that it

doesn't age you and trigger destructive chemical reactions in your body: just breathe deeply. In fact, you can turn it into a virtuous cycle with a productive response to any kind of stressful event.

The reason why deep and healthy breathing is so important is because it helps transport nitric oxide—a very potent lung and blood vessel dilator that resides in your nasal passages—to your lungs. So it makes your lungs and blood vessels function better. Taking deep breaths helps your lungs go from 98 percent saturation of oxygen to 100 percent oxygen saturation. Another benefit is that it helps improve the drainage of your lymphatic system, which removes toxins from your body. Of course, breathing deeply also helps in relieving stress. The deep breaths act as a mini-meditation and, from a longevity standpoint, are an important stress reliever. Shifting to slower breathing in times of tension can help calm you and allow you to perform at higher levels mentally and physically.

Learn how to self-soothe productively: twice a day, for five minutes, practice one of the five techniques below. You can also call on your own stress-busting technique, such as a cork crunch, in which you hold a wine cork in your mouth to help relax your jaw. I suggest you try all five breathing techniques to find the one that allows events to energize you positively rather than negatively.

1. Diaphragmatic Breathing

Most people breathe the way they dance: they think they know what they're doing, but they don't have a clue. (I'll admit that free-form inspired dance has the benefit of being fun; just please keep the free-style breathing to a minimum.) Stop right now for a second and focus on your breathing. Now look down. See anything moving? Probably not. That's because most people typically take very short, shallow breaths—the kind that come from your chest. For you to really improve your lung function, you need to practice taking deep, whole breaths. Remember what makes the lungs move? Your diaphragm. That's the flat, dome-shaped muscle that contracts to expand your lungs and draw in oxygen.

To really learn proper breathing technique, it's a good idea to take yoga lessons. In yoga, people focus as much on their breathing as on their eventual ability to scratch their heads with their toes. But for now, try this exercise:

Lie flat on the floor, with one hand on your belly and one hand on your chest.

Take a deep breath, slowly. When you first practice, lying on the floor is important, because if you stand up, you're more likely to fake a deep breath by doing an exaggerated chest extension rather than letting it fill up naturally. Imagine your lungs filling up with air; it should take about five seconds to inhale. Your diaphragm expands your lungs as you take that breath in, and your belly button should be moving away from your spine as you fill your lungs. Your chest will also expand—and maybe rise ever so slightly—as you inhale.

When your lungs feel fuller than a sumo wrestler's lunch box, exhale slowly, taking about seven seconds to let out all the air. You can pull your belly button toward your spine to force all the air out of your lungs. Take ten deep breaths in the morning, ten at night, and as many as you need when shooting free throws or after chasing your toddler down the cereal aisle.

2. Breathing Exercise 4 by 4

Take a slow, deep diaphragmatic breath followed by a normal breath, and repeat four times. Do these eight breaths four times a day or whenever you need to self-soothe. You can even practice at a red light, standing in a line, waiting on the phone, before a meeting, after an event that could be stressful to you, or when you are about to say something you know you'll wish you hadn't.

3. Nose-Inhale, Mouth-Exhale Breathing

In this pattern, you do exactly what it says. Inhale a diaphragmatic breath through your nose, hold for a count of five, and then exhale through your mouth; just let your jaw drop, as though you are letting the breath escape. The exhale should take two to three times as long as the inhale.

4. Focus on Your Space Breath

Focus on the pause between one of your breaths out—your exhale—and the next breath in. It is the little pause of quiet and stillness. Take the next inhaled diaphragmatic breath when you are ready and avoid holding your breath. Your exhale should take twice as long as your inhale. As you become more comfortable and calm, you will be able to stay in the pause space longer. Let yourself enjoy this calm and quiet space.

5. Guided Imagery Breathing

Guided imagery isn't the screen of your car's GPS; it is really purposeful dreaming, putting your imagination to its best use. The technique has been shown to improve mood, ease depression, and decrease stress. How do you do it? Go to a quiet place—the bathroom often works well, since privacy is usually respected there. Start by relaxing and breathing deeply, and then visualize yourself in different scenarios. Some variations include imagining yourself in a pleasant place (the beach), fighting disease (seeing your good immune cells fighting off bad germs), and practicing for a big performance (doing well in your job). Here's an example of how guided imagery can cure aches and pains: if you're in pain, visualize the spot of pain. Follow the nerve from that spot to the center of your mind. Ask your body if you can take control of that pain, and visualize the way that would happen.

Try out all of these techniques. You shouldn't, however, have to limit yourself to any one technique. The point is for you to find what works best for you. This is actually one of the reasons why the buddy system is so important: the one-on-one relationship is a natural stress reliever. And having someone you trust—who you can vent to or talk through problems with—provides a sense of calm, helps put things in perspective, and even gives you that push to stop procrastinating over your particular stressor. Other people turn to activities like writing in a journal or doing yoga or some other form of physical-mental activity that quiets the stress response. I wish I could tell you the one thing that works, but that's really the whole point: I can't tell you what will work for you. But you can.

#4 | Know What Kind of Stress You're Dealing With

Most of us probably divide stress into two categories: that which will make you tear your hair out and that which will make you want to wallop somebody in the lip. Fear and frustration and anger. While it's true that much of your stress feels the same way (blood boiling), the truth is that there are actually different kinds of stressful events, and your body knows this. The events that you typically don't have to worry about over the long term are the acute kind: the stress happens right in front of you, but you know that there is an end and a solution in sight. Maybe it's the person who cuts you off on the highway: you're mad, but you're generally over it in a few minutes. Or maybe it's something serious like breaking a leg: You're stressed because of the pain and the problems it may cause, but you also know that time will typically heal you and you'll eventually return to your normal state. That's not to say that those kinds of events don't cause a stress response or aren't harmful to your body, but they generally aren't as problematic over the long term.

The two categories of stress that really are the body barrag-

232

ers are the ones that nag chronically and the ones that are major life events. The nagging stressors may seem small, but they chip away at you, because you can't seem to get those tasks taken care of and forgotten. Think of a hoarder's home: a little stuff accumulates, and then a little more, and then more and more and more, until one day you can't even walk through the house without climbing over boxes and twelve-day-old bowls of chili. You want to get that closet cleaned out, but you put it off again and again—until just the very thought of it seems overwhelming. That's how those nagging stresses work: they just pummel you at low levels until your body is regularly in that chronic state of elevated stress response. Heck, that's what's sapping the life out of our nurses throughout America: that repeated wait as they log onto their computer for each patient. Even if the stressor seems minor, the fact that it's never resolved gradually breaks down the body.

But you can beat this type of stress. One of the most powerful examples I've seen concerned a patient of mine who had the autoimmune skin condition psoriasis, as well as arthritis. She also suffered from insomnia (and sleep problems for the better part of ten years). One of her docs wanted to put her on the three most powerful anti-immune disease medications. But get this: she learned how to meditate and to live in the moment, and she was able to control the nagging stress of her chronic conditions so well that she didn't even need the medications. She eliminated the symptoms that came from her arthritis, and she got her sleeping back on track. All within ten days. Incredible. Yes, psoriasis varies in severity from time to time, but when she stops meditating it comes back; when she resumes she gets rid of it. While I think all can benefit from stress management, do not stop your medications without your doc working with you and agreeing to monitor you. See, preventing the arthritis caused by psoriasis early on is important to maintain long-term joint function.

The other category of stress is major life events such as a death in the family, a move, a divorce. They may cause conflict or angst—long-term or short-term—but they're so major that you know that they're going to change your life for at least two years. Yes, that is how long it typically takes for the pain from a major life event to fade. With those major events, there often *isn't* a solution, which is why "solving the problem" doesn't work all the time. You can't always find a solution when a divorce is at stake, and you certainly can't reverse a death in the family. It's been shown that these major life events can age us by more than two years automatically, and there's no denying that when faced with these kinds of stressors, you do need to employ strategies that relieve the stress response or raise dopamine and oxytocin levels to mitigate the effects. While yoga won't change your life situations, it will help calm your body and mind. That is what we're after. Incorporating one or more favorite stress management techniques into your life will help you to better meet the twists and turns of life (and do your Do-Over).

Researchers have actually determined which life events produce the most stress. In the 1960s, doctors Richard Rahe and Thomas Holmes studied five thousand medical patients to create a stress scale as a predictor of illness. Using their calculations, they determined these were the events or situations with the highest stress scores and their likelihood of contributing to illness.

Death of a spouse	100
Divorce	73
Marital separation	65
Imprisonment	63
Death of a close family member	63
Personal injury or illness	53
Marriage	50
Dismissal from work	47
Marital reconciliation	45
Retirement	45
Change in health of family member	44
Pregnancy	40
Sexual difficulties	39
Gaining a new family member	39
Business readjustment	39
Change in financial state	38
Death of a close friend	37
Change to a different line of work	36
Change in frequency of arguments	35
Major mortgage payments that cause worry	32
Foreclosure of mortgage or loan	30
Change in responsibilities at work	29
Child leaving home	29
Trouble with in-laws	29
Outstanding personal achievement	28
Spouse starts or stops work	26
Beginning or end of school	26
Change in living conditions	25
Revision of personal habits	24
Trouble with boss	23
Change in working hours or conditions	20
Change in residence	20

Change in schools	20
Change in recreation	19
Change in church activities	19
Change in social activities	18
Minor mortgage or loan	17
Change in sleeping habits	16
Change in number of family reunions	15
Change in eating habits	15
Vacation	13
Christmas	12
Minor violation of law	11

Holmes-Rahe Social Readjustment Rating Scale (Holmes and Rahe, 1967)

Score of 300 or higher: at risk of illness.

Score of 150 to 299: risk of illness is moderate
(reduced by 30 percent from the above risk).

Score of less than 150: slight risk of illness.

Now, I will say that one of the major life events that seems to affect so many people—and does have solutions—involves financial problems. It has become one of our top stressors as a nation and even as a world population, as more and more people accumulate more and more debt and are getting themselves into some real financial trouble. So I can say that every person looking for a health Do-Over should also do a wealth Do-Over: that is, take a good, hard look at your financial situation and make any adjustments necessary to ensure financial security, even if that means bringing in personal wealth and money-management experts to help you do so. If you don't get you finances in check, your body may soon follow down that same path of insolvency—leading to a double whammy of destruction.

While my expertise is certainly not giving financial advice, I can tell you that, according to research, the stress over finances is destructive to health and to relationships. It's often listed as one of the top reasons why marriages fail. So getting your financial life in order is imperative. Furthermore, some of the best financial strategies my patients have used to help straighten out this part of their lives are ones that any of us can follow, like paying yourself first. For example, put 10 percent of your earnings toward savings to help build investments, allocating emergency accounts, and giving yourself a safety net. Another plan is to make specific budgets and then stick to them. After all, many people use shopping the same way that others use eating: as a way to temporarily ease stress, even though it may have a destructive outcome. That new purse or watch might be nice for a moment, but it will only add to your stress level if you're living beyond your means. One way to think about money problems is to equate it to eating issues: Overspending is like overeating; the choices you make today may feel good in the short term, but they have very severe consequences in the long term. They're not always easy to address, but creating systems like the ones I mentioned above— and slowly chipping away at the big problem—is the way that you can get your financial situation straightened out. Just like you can't lose fifty pounds in a weekend, you can't erase debt in one paycheck. But small changes over time—more walking and less sugar; more saving and less spending—build up to eventually get you to the place where you want to be.

#5 | Caregivers Need Care, Too

The reality is that one of the greatest stresses we have is caregiver stress—that is, the feeling that we're responsible for others. Stress is really the price of caregiving. That can come in any form: caring for others financially, logistically, emotionally, and when those close to you have health problems.

Maybe it's like sympathy-pregnancy pains, in a way. You hurt when you feel others around you are hurting, and you feel helpless if you cannot relieve some of their pain. That caregiver stress is not only a nagging one but also a major one, giving you a two-sided challenge to trying to relieve stress. Now, we all know that the most bubblicious bath in the world won't do a darn thing to ease the ongoing tension that comes with caregiver stress, so you shouldn't pretend that it will unless you combine it with some other form of stress management. The best you can hope for is to incorporate all of your stress management tools: (1) use small strategies to help get little spritzes of dopamine to take the edge off when you can, and (2) do what you can to try to solve the problem at hand, whether it's being more proactive about the health of the person you're caring for, getting help for financial woes, or any other concern that's weighing you down.

I've seen this firsthand so many times, including one nurse who had to care not only for her own patients but also for her sister who had cancers of the brain and ovary. What's more, she had kids at home, too. The feeling of guilt was overwhelming, as was the stress of trying to handle all of her responsibilities. Her way of coping was to tackle the tasks head-on by creating a Google calendar that her family could use and share so that everyone could contribute to caregiving with easy and efficient communication. The situation ended up bringing the family closer together.

Guilt, of course, is one of the biggest and least productive forms of internal stress. Caregivers are often anticipating loss (worse stress-wise than actual loss), and it's not atypical to imagine at some level the relief that could come with losing the person they're caring for. This thought can trigger strong feelings of guilt on top of already complicated emotions of sadness and loss. Additionally, caregivers are often also coping with resentment—another stress ager that doesn't net a person anything but more of the stress hormone cortisol—perhaps because siblings, spouses, or others aren't helping to the extent they think they should be. Or maybe there's a combination of a lot of different feelings, especially because health caregivers are unable to address effectively their loved ones' pain or illness.

I think of many caregivers as having "carrying-the-world-on-your-shoulders" syndrome. Well-meaning caregivers often believe they are the only ones who can take good care of their loved one. This is a mistake. It takes a village to care for a disabled or elderly parent, and it takes a community of social support to care for a caregiver. It is not caregiving that causes stress, but rather the sense of burden and loss that often accompanies it. Having help is essential to enjoying and honoring what is often the final stage of a loved one's life. Giving yourself room for your own pain and being willing to accept support from others is key to supporting a person as he or she transitions. These are not easy issues to handle, grapple with, and deal with fully—especially while going through both the logistics and the emotions that caregivers do. So perhaps the greatest advice that I can give all types of caregivers is the one I started the book with: partner up. Not just to count calories and go for walks, but to know whom to lean on when you need it the most.

#6 | Lust the List

We all know how it feels when our brains are swirling with overload: so much to do, so much to think about. We have the untouched piles of forms for our two kids' schools, the rescheduled doctor's appointment that we absolutely cannot miss, not to mention all of our work stuff, and then we can't forget Aunt Marge's ninetieth birthday, and then this, that, this, that, more more more more more—it never ends. You feel like your brain is a neurological jambalaya overflowing with ingredients. That overwhelming swirling sensation is what causes you stress.

But here's what I think. I think most people are equipped to handle lots of tasks. You can do a lot. You *do* do a lot. And you can do them all well, even if you're pulled in more directions than a piece of gum stuck on the sidewalk. What causes you to have a stress response isn't *only* about the volume—though volume does contribute to stress, and many people don't know how to say no. A stress response occurs when you are overwhelmed trying to keep it all straight—and to keep up with today's technology. While our technology is expanding its capacity exponentially, our human brains are not. The inability to keep up, especially in our 24/7, digitally connected world, is pretty darn stressful. We fear we'll forget something big. We know we have a lot of tasks, and we worry about how we'll fit them all in. And I contend that what causes *your* stress response is what you are telling yourself during all of the "doing," not the doing itself. Are you angry you have so much to do? Do you feel like you are helpless? Do you go to bed at night and focus on what you didn't get done, or do you pat yourself on the back for what you did accomplish? Is all the doing one continuous problem in your life?

Speaking anecdotally, I can tell you this: The more organized you are, the less stressed you are by an event, no matter how much you have on your plate. So whether your organizational tool comes in the form of a to-do list, a calendar, a reminder app, or a good old-fashioned pencil and paper, this is your ticket to adding control and decreasing anxiety. Now, I can't tell you which method you should use, because there are plenty of organizational tools, from analog to digital, out there, and personal preference should dictate your choice. But I can tell you that one part of stress management is really about thought and task management. Being organized is important to life being manageable, and keeping a schedule while still giving yourself room to roll with the punches—or adapt to the inevitable disruptions that will arise—will leave you feeling confident and settled even in unexpected situations.

The power of making a list is that it gives you the ability to see your entire day/week/month ahead so that you can prioritize what you need to do and when you need to do it by, and it allows you to unplug fully when you have scheduled yourself to unplug and to really focus when you're working. That list eliminates the angst we all have of forgetting to do something, and it gives you the power to prioritize—and even delegate if you can't get to things. Most of us don't want to abdicate responsibility. We want to relieve the tension that comes from wondering whether we can get it all done. When we feel that our responsibilities are manageable, the result is that we get to relax and be more present in our moment-to-moment life as it's happening, knowing that we've set a time to take care of what's next. Just remember to schedule time for you to schedule your time.

It's really the same concept that works in other areas of your life. If you approach diet by the seat of your pants, you'll likely eat more junky food than you want. A lot more. But if you're organized and plan out your shopping to prepare healthy meals for you and yours, you have a much better shot of fueling your body with health-promoting, nutrient-rich foods. If you think your exercise routine is just going to come to you at eight thirty at night when you're already settled in on the couch watching a Netflix series, chances are you won't set out for a sweat session. But if you plan to hit ten thousand steps a day or schedule your workouts, you're more likely to get them in. Same holds true for your stress and responsibilities. With no organizational tools, you're constantly treading water—just hoping to keep afloat. But with tools that allow you to methodically add and subtract tasks, you'll swim strong through your day and cover a heck of a lot of ground in the process.

#7 | Unplug (But Not All the Way)

There's no question that we live in a time when we're tethered to our technology. You need your phone(s) the way you need air, food, and a sharp toenail clipper. You crave feeling connected to your friends, to your work, to the world, and you do that through email, social media, and—by gosh— even some old-fashioned talking to one another. Even though I'm no Clayton Kershaw, I'm going to throw you a curveball.

I'm not going to beg and plead with you to disconnect from the world. I'm not going to tell you the value of unplugging the technology and plugging into your senses and the earth around you. And I'm not going to tell you that technology, when it comes to making you unhealthy, is more evil than a chocolate lava cake. While there's certainly a case to be made that technology and the habits that go with it can be a source of stress, we can't just make a sweeping statement that eliminating the technology will eliminate the stress. Remember, the stress doesn't disappear just because you get away from it all. So what happens when you unplug for a good, long stretch? You worry about what may be awaiting you when you plug back in, you feel out of it, and you might even feel *more* stress being disconnected than you do when you're overconnected.

I will share an example from my own life. I was recently visiting a place where phones and technology weren't allowed. I went for five days, and when I returned, I had four thousand emails waiting for me. Really: four thousand. That doesn't help relieve stress, it adds to it. While I felt more relaxed after a few days without my tech, I can tell you that I felt anxious, worrying about patients and other responsibilities. De-teching doesn't always mean de-stressing.

I learned a few things about technology from that trip. First, at a practical level, I can put an out-of-office reply on my email: "Sorry, I will not be able to respond to this. Please email me again in one week." And I also learned that just because something is techy doesn't mean I have to think of it as being "bad." The trick—and this is different for everyone—is that you have to find the sweet spot where you can balance both. Can you find a way to stay semiconnected when you're disconnected on a vacation or a family outing? Maybe it's promising to check email for only thirty minutes in the morning. Maybe it's just sneaking a peak at your phone while everyone else is taking showers. Maybe it's making a deal with your family that if you can have two hours a day to work, the rest of your hours will be 100 percent theirs. Or maybe it is taking that week or weekend with no tech at all. That's okay too.

What you're after: finding that time in your life where you can take some time for yourself while not creating even more stress and anxiety as a result of being away from your work. After all, vacation doesn't mean that the problems disappear. Knowledge, in fact, is a great stress reliever. So as long as you know that everything is under control, it is possible to experience peace even knowing you will return to your task list at some later scheduled time. It's when you don't know what's waiting for you—or when you feel you have no control over what might be waiting for you—that you feel the most angst.

So my advice to you when you're trying to get away is this: Make a deal. Make a deal with yourself, and make a deal with your family. Find the least amount of technology drip you need and then stick to your plan. If you need some time to handle the occasional emergency, fine. Remember, your goal isn't to eliminate stressful events, it's to manage your response to them and not let your stress response get the best of you. That's the point when your Do-Over becomes sustainable: when it is integrated in a way that empowers you in all areas of your life.

Love in Your Life

7 Things You Need to Know
About Sex and Relationships

When it comes to your Do-Over, there's no question as to what the most important room of your house is: your kitchen. Of all actions you can take, it's the choices you make about what foods you do or do not eat that tell all those little and big chemical processes in your body whether they should be working or malfunctioning, whether they should be burning fat or storing it, and whether you should have lots of energy or too little of it. Food, as you know by now, is really what moves the needle—for better or worse.

But I want to talk about the other thing we associate with the phrase "for better or worse"—that is, your relationships, and, more specifically, what happens in another room in your house: the bedroom. Granted, I fully recognize that you're not limited to only the bedroom, and if having a romantic interlude on the washing machine, on the stairs, or in the coat closet is your thing, then by all means, go for it. After all, it is the unexpected and the risky that fire up

247

the dopamine that can keep sex hotter than it was at age twenty-five.

Yup, part of getting your Do-Over means doing the deed.

Why? Because the data show that having sex in a loving and monogamous relationship has a profound effect on longevity and overall health. The more and better sex you have, the longer and happier you live. (Yes, I love to write prescriptions: "Sex, as hot as possible, every morning, or at least three times a week." As some of my patients, female and male, say, "Sign me up, Doc!")

Easy to write, but not as simple to do. It's not as if one walks up to his or her partner and orders up a healthy dose of sex the way someone orders the grilled chicken salad instead of the fried chicken parmesan. "Yes, honey, I'd like to start with an appetizer of extended kissing, and then for the main course, I'd like twelve minutes of missionary, followed by a warm cuddle as we drift off to sleep. Sure, why not, throw in a side order of whipped cream!" Though, heck, maybe it ought to be that way sometimes.

Why do I say that? Because in this society, we have some serious hang-ups and roadblocks when it comes to making sure that we have regular and high-quality sex in our relationships. It can be complicated, I know, because sex isn't about sex. Sex is about everything that happens in our worlds before and after sex. It's about how we treat each other, how we talk to each other, how we fight with each other. It's not *really* about lingerie and toys and satin sheets. Sex, most times, is about everything but the sex.

So to get your Do-Over in life, it may also mean getting a Do-Over in your sex life, too.

In this chapter, I'm going to take you through the seven key principles for improving your relationships and the sex that you have. After all, who doesn't want better sex and an honest and open relationship? Not just for peace of mind but for a healthy body, too. Just do me one favor: don't read this chapter in bed. You should be saving that space for something else.

#1 | Know Your Most Potent Sex Organ

Oftentimes middle school health class is where we learn all the basic biology about how our bodies work—specifically, what part goes into what part, with the outcome of extending the survival of our species. (Unless it was the naughty neighborhood kid who took you behind the alley and told you about how men and women make babies.) For kids, that's a necessary part of the process: learning how our bodies are supposed to function. And I'm not condemning sex-ed classes for doing this dutiful job, but I also want to point out that too often sex-ed classes seem like they're making the case that sex is about plugs and sockets, in and out, penis and vagina—that sex is about what goes on below the belt.

That, we know, is 100 percent biologically true. Can't make babies without plugs or sockets. But I also think that we take that truism and hold onto it as if this law of biology is the only sexual scientific fact there is. The real truth is—

especially when you grow older and your hormones aren't the only things that make your primal sexual decisions—that the more important relationship isn't groin to groin. It's brain to brain.

Perhaps the most potent chemical involved in the matter of love is oxytocin, the bonding hormone that's stimulated to secrete from your brain when you bond with someone. It, like the neurotransmitters dopamine and serotonin, is a feel-good chemical, so when we're attracted to another person, when we're in a healthy relationship with another person, and when we touch another person, the oxytocin flushes through our system. And we feel good. It's why sex feels good (well, one of the reasons why sex feels good), and it's why love feels good. So ultimately, this is what we're after as bonding creatures: being in a relationship that continually stimulates the release of oxytocin.

There is, however, a biological catch. Oxytocin, while stimulating arousal in both genders, manifests itself in different ways in men and women; hence the whole Mars-Venus debate. In men, when oxytocin rises, it tends to heighten arousal. And in women, oxytocin decreases the stress hormone cortisol—meaning that love allows women to focus by reducing stress and anxiety and increasing a feeling of security. You can see how these factors, while both beneficial, could be at odds. When men feel the bond, they get va-va-voom excited, while women tend to calm. Does that mean we can't be compatible sexually because of our biology? Of course not. It just helps to realize that the way we bond together may exhibit itself differently.

Now, why is this so important? Because those couples

with the highest oxytocin levels are the ones with the highest rates of longevity. See? It's healthier to be happier. This happiness level (the bonding level, in essence) stems only partly from how many times you have sex or whether you know how to experiment in the bedroom with ice cubes, Jell-O, or blindfolds. Many other shared activities stimulate oxytocin: talking to each other, sharing with each other, hugging, kissing each other hello and good-bye, complimenting each other. Those are all things that happen with your cerebral parts, not your private parts.

When you share bonding moments, this causes your brain to release oxytocin. In turn, oxytocin stimulates the parts of the brain that control sexual arousal: the cingulate and the insula. So it all works together. When you combine the oxytocin factor with the fact that the brain is responsible for your emotions (through the almond-shaped amygdala, pronounced a-*mig*-da-la), arousal, attraction, and so many other things when it comes to matters of love, you realize that perhaps we've spent way too much time trying to solve sexual dysfunction by repairing the parts rather than looking at the master control board.

#2 | Sexual Function Is Not as Much About Parts as It Is About Pipes

Now, you know that your brain is the primary influencer of the quality of your sex, but I would be remiss if I didn't address the fact that sometimes our machines do break down, sometimes our parts don't work, and sometimes it is the sex organs that do not function properly. (We want to have sex, but it's not all that easy.) That kind of work does require some fixing, but I'd also argue that oftentimes we're looking in the wrong place.

Our bodies are not like cars. If your car has a flat tire, you inspect the tire, look for the nail, remove the nail, plug the puncture hole, and you're on your merry way. If you—sexually (and obviously metaphorically)—have a flat tire, the first place you should inspect isn't your actual tire. Yes, we can treat sexual dysfunction with meds, lubes, and pumps; some cases do require those kinds of fixes. But when it comes to sexual dysfunction, we need to spend more time looking under the hood. That's because the number one thing that causes sexual dysfunction is the number one thing that will cause total-body dysfunction: bad blood flow caused by inflammation. The two major factors that determine whether a sexually active couple at age fifty-eight will still be having sex at age eighty-five are: one, if both partners are still alive and the couple is together; and two, the level of inflammation the man has in his system at age fifty-eight. Yes that is real (and really robust) data from a major US study, the National Social Life, Health, and Aging Project.

While hormones and other chemical processes certainly influence your desire to have sex, your ability to have quality sex is dictated by blood flow: that is, how well blood moves through your arteries to your penis or vagina. For men to have an erection, blood needs to flow freely through the arteries into the penis; the blood is subsequently trapped there in order to maintain the erection. And for women, proper blood flow is important to help stimulate nerve endings and lubrication, both important factors for pleasure and orgasm. So what's that mean? Many of the reasons why our parts don't work correctly is because the blood is getting diverted or slowed down somewhere along the circulatory transit system. That could be caused by conditions such as diabetes, high lousy LDL cholesterol, and high blood pressure, all of which mess up the in-and-out flow of blood through the body. Now, a gas you put out—no, not that kind of gas—is key here. Nitric oxide is made by the endothelial cells lining your arteries. This gas is the same gas whose effect is prolonged by erectile dysfunction drugs like Viagra and Cialis. Nitric oxide gas dilates your arteries, and you produce two types of it: an "always there" source that causes fast dilation and, in the context of exercise, enables you to run fast without much of a warm-up. Then there is the kind that lets you run longer and harder after your warm-up. In fact, as we get older, we need to warm up longer on the track and in bed, too, as our always-there nitric oxide fades, leaving just the type of nitric oxide that we must activate with our own warm-up. This is one of the reasons why we need that warm-up period in bed: to open up the blood vessels to allow blood to flow freely to our erogenous zones to help us have sexual satisfaction.

So this may sound like the least sexy of suggestions, but it's the truth: if you want to have better sex, eat vegetables. If you want to have better sex, walk ten thousand steps a day. If you want to have better sex, you need to manage your responses to stressors. If you want to have better sex, eat more healthy fats. If you want to have better sex, do what's good for your entire cardiovascular system.

This, folks, is the real reason why sex is truly a matter of the heart.

#3 | More Sex, Better Sex = Longer Life

One thing we haven't discussed much here is the difference between certain kinds of scientific studies. That's a major part of the scientific world: not just collecting the data points, but getting at the crux of how the data were gathered and what the data mean. For example, there's a big difference between studies that clearly show cause and effect—such as those animal studies where you can control all factors except the ones you're studying—and ones that demonstrate *relationships* between two factors. In the latter kind of study, we can't say x causes y, but we can say that two factors are related. These are often epidemiologic studies: studies in which we gather a large sample of population data (age, gender) and lifestyle data (eating habits, sexual habits). When you analyze that data, you can come up with relationships; for instance, people who eat more vegetables per day have less inflammation and live longer. Do we know that eating vegetables causes these changes in inflammation and longevity? Maybe not in this kind of example, not in a cause-and-effect way, but we know there's a link.

Such is the case with studies investigating longevity and

sex and orgasms. We can't do typical cause-and-effect studies in this area because there'd be no way to prove that the
mechanism between having lots of good sex causes your
heart to beat *x* amount of years "younger" (as if you had the
energy and health of someone much younger) than it would
if you didn't have sex. But we can conduct these epidemiologic studies where we look at the relationship between two
factors: comparing sexual quantity and quality with longevity. These studies have a lot of value because they can focus
on factors that may not be able to be studied in other ways,
and they allow us to track data over long periods of time.

Okay, so I know all this chatter about study mechanics is
about as sexy as a cinder block, but I do think it's important
to realize the context of how some science is carried out, so
you can understand the big picture. I can't prescribe you a
three-times-a-week mandate of sex and say that it will clear
up your blues in seven to ten days the way I can prescribe a
lung-infection-and-cough medication. But I can give you
that same prescription and tell you that the data indicate
you'll be better off for it in the long run because of it.

Here's some of the research: older studies show that the
more orgasms a man has, the less likely he is to develop
prostate cancer. And frequent orgasms for women appear to
extend their longevity for a variety of reasons. According to
data from the late 1990s in Great Britain, and from the con-
temporary National Social Life, Health, and Aging Project
I mentioned before, a man who has one orgasm a week and
increases that to three times a week decreases his risk of dying
by about 20 percent. And if he increases it to one a day, or
about 350 a year, he decreases the risk by about 40 percent.

There aren't enough data on women to link frequency to longevity, but quality of sex in both Great Britain and the United States correlates positively with better health for women.

Now, we don't completely know the mechanism that's at play, though the data indicate that orgasms from either a healthy relationship or masturbation are okay, while there isn't as much of an effect from unhealthy relationships. There is speculation that sex has an effect on stress levels, so when there's a close bond between two people, sex reduces stress responses for both men and women. Sex in that healthy relationship enables them to handle major life stresses much more effectively than they would having sex in an unhealthy relationship—one that's filled with all kinds of stresses for other reasons.

One patient of mine, Robert, was literally addicted to food. Ate a lot, ate frequently, almost ate himself to death. He had read in one of my previous books that sex is a craving that's located in the same part of the brain as other crave centers (for food, thirst, and sleep), and that one of the ways to beat back a food addiction is to see if you can satisfy that craving with some other craving, including sex.

So he talked to his wife, explained that he wanted to get healthy, and that—by goodness!—he had the answer: frequent sex!

Now, you may think this was simply some ploy for Robert to have more sex, but his wife was interested, wanted to help, and she agreed to give it a go. So they had sex—a lot of sex. After the first two months, he lost 14 pounds. It seemed to be working, so they kept on going, often having sex multiple times a day. (Robert's wife was his true buddy!)

The result: Robert lost 140 pounds. I repeat: Robert lost 140 pounds. And he has kept it off.

While not the only change that he made, frequent sex made Robert healthier—and saved his life. I should note that it's obviously important that you have a partner who matches your sexual appetite. I should also note that many of Robert's friends asked if his wife would talk to their wives. (Robert and his wife weren't invited over to as many friends' houses for get-togethers after that.)

Does Robert's story mean I'm advocating that you all go hibernate in the bedroom and buh-bump your way to a longer life? No, of course not. But I am suggesting that the healthier your relationship, the better your sex, and the better and more frequent your sex, the healthier and physiologically younger you'll be. And that's why perhaps the most important principle to follow in all of this is the next one.

#4 | After Initial Attraction, Relationship Success Hinges on One Thing

Maybe it's because of poems, songs, or romantic comedies, but for whatever reason, culturally we accept the notion that love stories should all end up in the same place: happily ever after. Though I guess between celebrity news and country songs, we should know this isn't true. Even still, when we enter most relationships, we're absolutely after the happily ever after. We dream of dancing the night away, of long walks in the woods, of crepes in Paris, of laughing and loving, of sipping coffee with a smile as the morning light shines just so on our relationship.

And then reality hits: The bills mount. The dishes are left undone (again). The baby won't sleep through the night. The potty-training child decides that the middle of the mall, on a day you forgot the diaper bag, is the perfect location for a geyser-like bout of diarrhea. The teenager has Instagram drama. Stress from work carries into the home. He said. She said. Fight, stress, anger, frustration—*aaaaaaah!*

When any or all of those doses of real life hit, we're left trying to manage the conflict, smooth the sea, and figure out how we're going to fix problems and prevent them from happening again.

And let's face it, that mall episode doesn't exactly get you in the mood—unless the mood is "tear your hair out in fistful clumps" mood.

So how do we make it all work? How do we strike the romantic ideal while still knowing that life isn't one big wine-filled walk down the Champs-Élysées?

Good questions, and I guess if we truly knew the answer, our national divorce rate wouldn't be 48 percent. Still, let me take a crack at it.

Biologically, we're attracted to other people through chemicals called pheromones—this is essentially what links us to other people via smells. (It's probably biology's way of making sure we don't mate with our cousins.) We don't know why we're attracted to some people and not others; it's simply an uncontrollable biological reaction.

My wife, Nancy, and I met in the ER. She was the pediatrician on call, and I was running the ER. The nurses hated me because I always infringed on their jobs and systems when I set up IVs before trauma patients came in, to make sure we were prepared for serious cases. So when word spread that I was interested in Nancy, the nurses told her, "Oh, no, don't go out with that Dr. Roizen!" Well, one day I did ask Nancy out with the oh-so-suave pickup line, "I just broke up after a relationship of seven years, and I'm depressed. Want to go out for a drink?" She said yes, we got married seven months later, and we've been married for forty-two wonderful years. Best thing I ever did. We got together because of our initial attraction—despite that horrible pickup line!—but we've stayed together because of other things we can control.

What you control is how far you're taking that attraction, assuming it's mutual—whether it's a lifetime, a year, a month, a date, a night, or a quickie in the hotel that charges by the minute. So how do you ensure a successful lifetime partnership? How do you know whether the attraction is worth making permanent? How do you know if it's right? I'd argue, and the data would support, that it's more than just a feeling of butterflies and tingles. It's actually the most crucial factor in determining whether you'll have a happy relationship and, by extension, a happy sex life.

It's a shared value system.

Specifically, for you to have relationship success, which I define as monogamous, low conflict, low stress, high sex, you need to have similar values when it comes to money, sex, and kids. When not in sync, those are the three things that tear apart marriages, and those are the three things that keep couples together when the two people are on the same page. So if you're at the stage where you're deciding on a life partner, well, you need to talk about these factors to make sure you have the same value systems when it comes to how you spend and save, how you want to raise your kids, and how often you want to have sex. Does that mean you have to be exactly the same? No. But if you're so far apart that you can't even talk about middle grounds, then you're simply destined to a lifetime of conflict and aches and stress—and by extension, very few intimate moments and very little sex. This means you have to get as granular and specific as possible to really feel out what your values and thoughts are when it comes to these three areas.

But what if you're already in your relationship and know that you're far apart where these three values are concerned? Admittedly, you're in a tough place, but your only strategy (assuming you want to save the relationship) is to talk things through and find areas where you can compromise. Bridging the gap in these values with maturity, mutual listening, and generosity will reduce the tension and stress that come from disagreements over such high-stakes subjects. You can even do a Do-Over to this part of your relationship.

In my relationship with Nancy, we rarely have conflicts, because we have that shared value system, but I remember one in particular we had over our children. I tried to make an argument about a particular learning program that I wanted our son and daughter to have. Nancy didn't think it would be ideal for our kids. But who was I to argue with Nancy, the pediatrician? And not just a pediatrician but a master developmental pediatrician and soon-to-be president of the Society of Developmental Pediatrics and co-author of the current reigning textbook in that field. As a matter of course, I deferred to her on all kids' medical issues, but on this one, I was convinced I was right. So we agreed— compromised—that we would ask an independent consultant her opinion. That person agreed with me—so we went to two more consultants, to be sure!

Another time, however, I wanted our young son to be able to go to a World Series game with one of our family friends. He had already missed school the previous year for a World Series game, and Nancy didn't want him to do it again. I used the line "But Nancy, it's a once-in-a-lifetime experience." She told me I had used that line last year. We compromised, and our son didn't go to the game. As it turns out, that was the night the big earthquake hit the Bay Area in the 1989 World Series, and Nancy and I were out of town, unable to reach people. I told her right then and there that I was grateful we didn't let Jeff go to the game. Two different scenarios—didn't matter who was right and who was wrong. It mattered that we listened to each other, respected the other person's opinion, and allowed for some give-and-take.

The only other real sticking point we had during our marriage was the amount of time I worked while we were on family vacations. We eventually worked out a schedule. I could work from three to eight o'clock in the morning, but then I would spend the rest of the time with the family, although I did nap in the afternoon. We came up with a system that satisfied everyone.

And we've done that throughout our marriage, with two

main rules: we never go to bed angry; and we never take opposite sides in front of the kids, working out disagreements in private. While our conflicts centered around kids and family, you can use the same principles to work through issues with money and sex: talk, compromise, work to figure out solutions.

The point of these stories isn't just to illustrate that compromise and civil discussion work; it's also that sometimes we're right and sometimes we're wrong, and to make a marriage work, you have to acknowledge that fact—and the fact that one person is no better or worse when things do or don't go his or her way. If you have those common values, and you're not 180 degrees apart on what you believe, it's much easier to close the gap when disagreements come up. Manage the conflict, ease the stress, live happier and healthier.

Easier said than done, you say. I gotcha. When you're in a relationship where there's a lot of conflict, it can feel like you're in an earthquake-rattled home: everything feels unstable, dishes are breaking, and it feels like your whole world is coming apart. And I can't sit here and say that with a snap of the finger and a few sage tips, you can work out every conflict. But I can tell you that disagreement in a relationship isn't about the actual thing you're arguing about; it's about a mind-set you take into a conflict. And the most productive and beneficial way you can be in a disagreement is to show respect for the other person's position and feelings and to spend more time listening than you do trying to persuade your partner that you are right. So I do think that most couples can work out most conflicts by following this approach to handling conflicts:

◆ Make your primary objective negotiation, not winning or losing. You'll both be happier in the long run if you don't treat the outcome of every argument like the result of a tennis match—because even when you "win," you lose. Instead, treat conflict a bit like buddy support that you should volley back and forth, talking through issues. When you do that, you're more likely to find common ground. Now, of course, there will be some situations where there's no middle ground—either you allow Junior to jump off the roof into the pool or you don't. (Please don't.) In those cases, you can still have a civil discussion, even if there are nonnegotiable issues at stake.

◆ Watch your tone and nonverbals. Much of the angst and tension that come from marital conflict don't happen because of the content of what you're fighting over but because of the tone in which things are said. Those subtle gestures—a condescending or cocky tone or an admonishing finger pointing—are what rattle the cage. So make a point to not only make your point, but do so with the same respect and thoughtfulness you'd extend to others. If you can do that, you've won half the battle. Respect each other's point of view and respect each other; that's the key, even if one of you is a liberal and the other from the Tea Party. (Happened to a successfully married couple we know.)

◆ Pause. There's no doubt that arguments can get heated. We can say things we don't want to say, that we don't mean, and that will send our relationships spiraling downward. Relationships are full of emotion and passion, and because of that, arguments can be, too. But it will do nobody any good if you argue in a "hot" state. What you want to do is remove yourselves from the situation— take deep breaths, take a walk around the block— and allow your stress response systems to calm and put you both in a more even-tempered or cerebral state. This change will allow you to do the first two strategies more easily. Now, be sure that you communicate what you're doing—that you're not trying to avoid the problem but rather trying to cool off so you can discuss it like adults.

#5 | Repeat After Me: No Shame

I think good health is a moral-free zone. I'm not here to preach or to judge or to ask you to change your beliefs. Healthy bodies aren't run by morality, they're run by biology. That perspective, as you know, is my training and profession. I do know that discussing sex and sexual topics can sometimes feel as if it's straying from the health zone to the personal-beliefs zone, and that's okay. You have to consider good health in the context of your own guiding principles.

That said, I think that too often a twelve-letter word has become a four-letter word. As a society (and a health care community), we don't talk about masturbation, we don't address masturbation, we don't even like to say "masturbation." And some of us don't even think it's okay to do it. But I hope we can, very soon, just get over it. Let's just get over the thought that if you masturbate, you're not happy and not healthy and not faithful.

Let me tell you the story of Nicole. She's married, had a couple of kids, but never really felt respect or warmth from her partner. Sadly, that's a common theme among many women I see. She never had an orgasm when she was younger, though she was pretty sure it was possible genetically, because her sister, as she described her, loved sex. Well, over time, Nicole gained weight and didn't feel loved—she never got hugged. So she bought a vibrator in hopes of getting some kind of sexual satisfaction. She didn't like it at all. When she came to me, she was ninety pounds overweight, and she confided in me about her sexual dissatisfaction. I told her that much of sexual pleasure is about blood flow, and if she wanted to increase her chances of orgasms, she had to lose weight, get in shape, and see what happened. Well, she lost ninety-four pounds, and she continued to use her vibrator; her husband had developed some dementia, and their relationship had turned asexual. Now she uses her vibrator often and enjoys her sex life. She told me recently, "My husband saw me after I lost the weight and called me a babe. It was the first time in my whole life he did that." Through the process, she gained respect for herself—and increased her own sexual pleasure by herself. The vibrator is good for her, it works for her, and it's making her healthier along the way.

My only caveat is this: this behavior is healthy as long

as you're not hurting your partner. This is also why shared values are important, so that your partner understands that masturbation isn't an indictment of a relationship. I'm all for anything that encourages health, relieves stress, and makes you happier. And if you have to steer the ship solo sometimes, then by all means, do so.

#6 | Little Investments Yield Big Results

If you put every penny that you find into a jar, it's going to take you a long, long (long, long, long, long, long) time before you build up enough capital to buy anything of any significance, be it a car, a house, or a new phone. And that's okay. There's nothing wrong with saving pennies to cash in on something later; it's just that you won't build up a whole lot of capital with minor investments.

Sex and relationships work the exact opposite way.

Pennies in equals millions out.

What do I mean by that? If you do the little things to make your relationship stronger, it will lead to huge outcomes of lower stress, better sex, and more longevity. Simple, really. The little-effort things that you can do for each other—all harkening back to what I talked about in point one, that your brain is your biggest sex organ—mean the greatest rates of return. That's why having great sex isn't about having more flexible hamstring muscles, investing in a trampoline for the bedroom, or taking strip-cardio classes. (No judgment if you do any of those things.) Great sex is about putting the pennies in the jar: finding the little yet lasting ways to make your partner feel good, feel wanted, feel satisfied. When you do that, your daily, weekly, yearly, and lifelong returns will turn those pennies into a sexual and soulful jackpot.

Some ideas:

◆ Give your spouse at least one compliment every day—and mean it. Make sure to include not only the things that the person can't control (such as appearance) but also things that require brain power (like decisions made, problems solved, or projects finished).

◆ Kiss on the cheek. Often.

◆ Plan a date. It gets harder and harder to find alone time, and sometimes it's necessary to carve out that time. After all, it's not necessarily the date itself that has to be quote-unquote romantic. It's the fact that you cared enough to want to spend the time together.

◆ Wash the dishes together. Sounds unromantic, but it gives you some quality talk time.

◆ Read the same book together and then talk about it, as long as you're reading at a similar pace. Intellectual stimulation leads to other kinds.

◆ Take a ten-minute walk together every day. Hold hands. Sometimes it's easier for men to have difficult discussions when they're side by side rather than face-to-face. This short habit could really improve communication.

#7 | You Should Always Have a Three-Way—with Dopamine!

I don't want to come across as pushing the point that sex is easy. It's not. Partners with different tastes and complicated lives and lagging energy and hormonal levels often have a hard time syncing up to make their sexual relationships satisfying and lasting. I know that for some couples, it can be hard to have sex once a week, once a month, once a year—and there are many reports of folks in nonsexual marriages who have sort of given up on the idea that they'll ever have sex with each other again. So I know there are roadblocks, and I do hope that the points I've covered in this chapter help you get over the hump so you can fully engage in your Do-Over, but I do know that it's not as easy as cleaning out your pantry and starting over with a new set of ingredients.

I do have to say that you need to come up with a tactic to make sure that you spark some romance, keep things fresh, and make sure that your relationships (sexually and emotionally) are always moving forward rather than stagnating like summer pond water. And the way you do it is with the one chemical we've talked about before: dopamine. Now, this neurotransmitter can be the source of some trouble because the need to increase dopamine is what causes unhealthy addictions. (Seeking the high we get from chips just causes us to want more chips to get that high all over again, so we need more and more chips to maintain those dopamine responses.) But what if we flip that principle in our favor so that we use dopamine to derive more and more pleasure from our relationships? That's when it all works. How do we do it? We do it in the same way that we do in other areas: we seek experiences that feel new, novel, and extraordinary.

So your job here isn't to swing from chandeliers as a form of foreplay, it's to make sure to integrate new and novel experiences into every part of your life. Don't get me wrong: habits are good and can be a strong means of establishing traditions. But your brain doesn't always want you to do the same thing every Saturday night. Your brain wants to go to dinner and a movie one night and then maybe try go-karts another time. Or moonlight hikes or walks through the neighborhood. Or plans with a couple you haven't seen in years. Or tasting parties like the kind I suggested in chapter 3. Just mix it up a little. If you want your engines running in the romantic area, then you have to work on keeping your whole system fresh, dynamic, and ready to go.

Passion Sense

7 Things You Need to Know
About Purpose in Life

When it comes to health and medicine, we live in a prescription-based world. You have strep throat? We prescribe penicillin. Overweight? We prescribe diet and exercise, and sometimes when you need a jump start or hit a plateau, we ask if you want diet pills with that. You gash your knee in a sidewalk fall? We cart you into surgery and repair that torn ligament. It took us a long time to get to this point, through studies, experiments, and advances in technology and thinking. There's a reason why science and medicine work the way they do. We want evidence that our methods of healing—and our methods of prevention—work for the majority of people who need it. Much of this book is based on these kinds of hard medical facts, repeat studies, and data that show when you do x, you get y. I've spent my whole life dealing with these kinds of equations that change and save people's lives.

I've also been in the health and wellness business (I hate

to call it that) for a long time. There's no doubt in my mind that while hard science is in the driver's seat when it comes to how we should prioritize our medical information, soft science should be a welcome guest in the passenger seat.

What do I mean by that? I know the term "soft science" is as loaded as Grandma's Thanksgiving Day table. Some will scoff at it, some will pooh-pooh it, some will think that soft science has zero credibility. And I get it. For some folks, if there's no clear, placebo-controlled evidence that a certain prescription works, then there's nothing to scientifically support that it's an effective tactic.

In my mind, however, soft science can have many meanings; and there's very good second-tier data that can offer insights into health and longevity. This chapter is about one of those areas: passion and purpose.

I can see why the science heads roll their eyes when the notion of passion comes up. After all, how do you measure passion with the precision with which you measure blood glucose? How can you see whether passion in your life opens up your arteries like some plaque-clearing drug? How do you systematically and repeatedly measure a burning desire the way you would track burning calories?

The first six Do-Over deeds you will be doing are all specific, concrete actions rooted deeply in biology and science. This last piece of your Do-Over is a little harder for science to quantify, but it's important in its own special way. It's the one that helps drive you to make good decisions; it's the one that motivates you day in and day out; it's the one that helps you relieve and manage stress (and those bad health outcomes that are associated with problematic responses to stressors); it's the one that gives you energy; it's the one that—frankly—makes it all worth it. Without further ado, let me announce your final Do-Over deed: to live your passion and find your purpose.

Now, I fully acknowledge that I can't prescribe you passion and purpose the way I can suggest you take a probiotic. Having passion for life and sensing a purpose for your life are states of mind that can't be defined and measured. I can't tell you what you like, what jazzes you, what gets you up and out in the morning.

#1 | The *Why* Is the Secret to It All

Here's why good health can be so hard for people: it's easy to be a sloth. Sit on the couch, watch *Wheel of Fortune* with a takeout quart of kung pao chicken, and then finish off with a bowl of ice cream the size of one of the Great Lakes. It's not always the easiest thing to make sure you have fish and vegetables and take those ten thousand steps and do all the little things that make you healthier and trigger the biological processes that kick-start your Do-Over. So many of us get into bad health situations because of this; it's easier to sit back than move forward. It's simple Newtonian physics: an object at rest will stay at rest unless propelled by an outside force. So when somebody tells us that we can reverse our habits with three apples, twenty minutes on the stair machine, four pills, and a frighteningly green kale smoothie every day, we think, "Oh my word, I don't have the energy to do all of *that*." And we revert to our Sajak-and-Vanna ways and have another quart of moo goo this or that.

So when you think about it, you realize that the real secret isn't *me* telling you what to do. It's you finding what makes it easier and more fun for *you* to make healthy choices because you want to. To do that, it's not about learning what makes your heart tick mechanically but what makes it beat deeply emotionally, psychologically. That really comes down to these two concepts:

Purpose in Life. This concept is exactly what you think it is: it's looking at your life and asking yourself why you're here. What do you uniquely contribute to your family, the community, the world? Sometimes passion and purpose are tied together like a braided ponytail, and sometimes they're not. I challenge you to think about this as you think about your Do-Over. Ask yourself not only what inspires you but also how you're helping others. When you acknowledge that you're serving a greater good, it's often much easier to have the rest of your life fall into place.

A compelling study from the University of Michigan illustrates exactly what I mean: when over seven thousand Americans above the age of fifty participated in an ongoing health survey measuring their sense of purpose in life, people with a powerful sense of purpose were more likely to maintain and achieve health and sign themselves up for screening exams like mammograms and colonoscopies than those with less purpose. Participants' sense of purpose was measured with questions they could agree with to a greater or lesser extent, such as: "I have a sense of direction and purpose in life," or "My daily activities often seem trivial and unimportant to me." The participants with higher purpose scores spent significantly less time at the hospital: the average time (seven nights over six years) dropped 17 percent for every point scored on the purpose scale. Regardless of whether a sense of purpose and health have a cause-and-effect relationship, being purposeful gives you drive to live life fully and perhaps drive to maintain your health—and that drive translates directly into cultivating your own well-being.

It's easy to be lazy and unhealthy when you don't have these driving forces serving as your psychological backbone to keep you all together. But once you have these two things straight in your life, it's actually easier to be healthy— because you're doing it for purposes bigger than your feelings, wants, complaints, or thoughts. You're doing it to have the energy to do what you love, and you're doing it because you feel good about helping others.

Always remember: the *why* in your life drives the *what you do* in your life.

Your Passion. What is it that excites you? What do you love doing? What would you do if you didn't get paid for it? Ideally, that can be your work, but it doesn't have to be. I'm fortunate enough to have two very strong passions. One is indeed my job of helping other people become healthy. I love it, absolutely love it. I can work nineteen hours a day on this and not feel as if I've worked a second—although afterward, I do need some sleep. In fact, I love deepening my understanding of prevention, reverse aging, and wellness so much that I take my medical literature to Cleveland Cavaliers basketball games to read during timeouts—to the point where my friends ask me if I'm crazy. I say, "No. I love it. I just love reading about medicine." You, too, may think I'm loonier than a tail-chasing kitty, but sorry, I get excited by jibber-jabber on how eliminating red meat cultivates bacteria inside you to prevent inflammation.

My second passion is squash—the sport, not the vegetable, though I do love the veggie, too. Love playing, love competing, love training, love the whole thing. Heck, after I retire from my day job, I may even try to win a national master's championship in the sport. Never once during all my years of playing did it ever feel like work, even when I was working hard and running stairs until I was ready to pass out.

I firmly believe that these two passions (plus my passions for Nancy and our kids) are big reasons why I've lived a healthy life. They're what drive me every day and inspire me to live the life that I want. Does that mean I don't have stress? Of course not. We all do. But doing what you love makes stressful events more manageable.

Your choice of passion doesn't matter. I don't care whether you like dancing or bird watching or fantasy football or Scrabble or knitting or photography or volunteering or baking or running or swimming or building computers or stamp collecting or antiquing or watching game shows from the 1970s. I care that you have *something*. For those of you who already know, live, and cultivate your passion,

I applaud you. And for those who don't carve out the time for it—or maybe haven't found it yet—I would prescribe this: make time to explore the world, try new things, experiment, get together with friends and family to see what it is that makes you feel like four million bucks. There is no need to get down in the doldrums because you don't think you have a passion or you think you've lost yours; you have license to explore, create, and discover that now. After all, even if you don't know where you're headed, your new journey will be a fun one.

#2 | You Can Game Your Biology

When we talk about passion and purpose, it would be easy to write off the concepts as touchy-feely areas of psychology. But I don't believe we should. The social sciences do explore and research these kinds of areas to help us understand how the brain and emotions work—and by extension, how we can use them to improve our lives and become healthier physically and mentally. I also think it would be a mistake to just write off passion and purpose as not having a biological basis, because certainly brain function is deeply rooted in biological and chemical relationships—influencing everything from decision making to emotional reactions and all of the things that affect how we make choices about our health. Who knows: someone might discover that passion and purpose change the bacteria in your gut so that it is easier to take your ten thousands steps a day, or reduce your blood sugar level. Right now it doesn't matter why passion and purpose affect your health decisions; what matters is that they do.

But to understand how passion and purpose can drive your Do-Over, it will help to know a bit of the current psychological science, especially when it comes to motivation. What is it that drives you to want to get healthy, stay healthy, make good decisions in the face of stress, and sustain your motivation? It's a good question, particularly when we live in a world full of temptations overflowing with cream, salt, and sugar.

Psychological theory says there are two kinds of motivation: extrinsic and intrinsic. The extrinsic kind, as you can guess, covers external factors. Intrinsic is obviously more of an internal kind of motivation. So let's take exercise as an example: having the motivation to go out and do four or five workouts a week, knowing that it takes some time to get into workout gear, perhaps drive to the gym, work hard and uncomfortably, shower, and then get back to it. What spurs you to go through all of that, when it's easier to have a piece of pie? Extrinsic motivation would be things like having some kind of bet with a coworker, or an employer reducing your health care premiums if your waist is less than half your height, or a set appointment every week with a trainer pushing you, or trying to fit into a wedding dress in six weeks— some outside force that gets you going. Intrinsic motivation would be, simply, that you exercise because you're called to do it, you love it, and you love the way you feel because of it. You might even hate putting on your sneakers or waking up early on those days when you know you won't have time in the evening, but you do it because what you get out of exercising is greater than whatever annoyances you step over to get there. You do it for the sake of exercise itself—and for that internal satisfaction, that feeling of strength or health that you get that inspires you to do it again and again and again. A self-regulating motivation, if you will.

Many experts argue that extrinsic motivation will fade, and you really need the intrinsic kind if you have any shot of developing lifelong habits. It's not enough to have the bet, because what happens when the bet is over? You need, the experts would say, a deeper meaning to gut out a forty-five-minute run in the park, or whatever your exercise mode of choice.

Here's where I disagree—but just a bit. While intrinsic motivation is the goal, we can't just whip up a case of intrinsic motivation and hope that it catches on and that we live our life with deep feelings of joy whenever we eat a plain celery stick. However, we can game the biology—trick our intrinsic systems—by using extrinsic motivations. You can take jumper cables to your motivational systems by using extrinsic methods to find your passion, to find what makes you inspired, to find what gets you going. If it's a photo of your former self on the fridge, so be it. If it's a weight-loss bet with your sister, go for it. If it's some other kind, that's okay too. The point is that you're outsmarting your reptilian brain and reaching a higher level of thinking. You're doing a few things to get you going and help you explore new habits, and then using those practices to catapult you to a now self-generated desire to continue them.

How so? Let's say that you have a weight-loss bet or are trying to lose weight before going on a beach vacation. Knowing that, and keeping that in the front of your mind, will be enough to help you make healthy decisions. The veggie sticks instead of the Oreos. The water instead of the soda. The blueberry instead of the blueberry pie. Once you start making those decisions, you start to feel better, look better, and be healthier. At some point, you start to transition to where the feeling, looking, and being serve as the intrinsic motivation more than the fleeting gratification of sneering, "I'm going to beat the mucus out of Kelly when we weigh in next week!"

Jennifer, a participant in my Enforcer eCoaching program, discovered this for herself when she adopted the practices of the Do-Over. Jennifer was sixty pounds overweight, hypertensive, and diabetic. She was a smart, willful woman, and when her employer provided a hefty extrinsic motivation to take on her health—a $400 reduction in insurance premiums for participating in our Enforcer eCoaching— she initially balked. She was annoyed. Jennifer didn't want to change her habits—a conclusion I made early on when I received her first email to me after an initial coaching exchange: a giant image of a finger. And not her ring finger.

Well, Jennifer put aside her negative feelings about the program and followed the coaching she received. She used this coaching program—independent of her employer but paid for by her employer (that employer really cares about its employees)—as her buddy. Ten months later, I got another email from her: "You know, I was mad as hell about being forced to do this. Turns out to be the best thing I've done for myself in years." Jennifer lost forty-seven pounds, got rid of her high blood pressure and type 2 diabetes, and has chosen to continue working with a buddy—in this case, her coach—to support her in creating new health goals. And though, of course, no one actually forced her to enroll, the extrinsic motivator of the insurance premium discount was so compelling that she felt she could not pass it up. What she got as a result was not only a Do-Over but also an ongoing internal resolve and drive to take on her health moving into the future.

Is there any guarantee that you will get lasting motivation from goals and targets? Of course not. But the fact is that 96 percent of Americans entering Medicare today (and 99 percent of Swedes; the only two countries for which we have solid data) simply do not have enough intrinsic motivation to launch an effective counterattack against our society's addictions and temptations (otherwise, we wouldn't have the obesity and other chronic disease stats that we have). In fact, only 4 percent of Americans take all the actions necessary to get that Do-Over, despite evidence that doing them drastically reduces the risk of adverse health events and premature death.

I'd argue that using extrinsic motivation is one of the most powerful ways to find the things that will give you lasting motivation. Motivational experts have identified the three ingredients for making motivation lasting: (1) autonomy (you have control and power over what you do), (2) competence (you show some sort of skill at whatever it is—and you hardly need that for a health Do-Over, except for walking, reading, and breathing), and (3) community (you have a support network to share in your ups and downs;

remember reading about this in chapter 1?). So when you're exploring a new passion or purpose, it will most likely come when all three of those elements are in place.

#3 | You Have to Be Open to All Possibilities

If you've read this far and you're wallowing in pity because you think you don't have a passion, or you've lost yours, or you're just stuck thinking about what you want to do with your life, then I know you may feel more frustrated than a driver in LA rush hour traffic. And I wish—how I wish— you could walk up to some store and order up passion the way you order up a coffee. "Yes, I'd like a double-shot of inspiration with a side of *woo-hoo! Extra large!*"

I feel your frustration, and I also wish I could offer you a surefire way to figure it out. But there's really only one answer: try this, try that, try this, try that. You have to be open to the notion that something you never dreamed of liking could be the very thing that changes your life. I have two patients who come to mind here. One man, a retiree, had lost his wife and was extremely depressed. He had enough money to live on but asked me for advice. Knowing what I knew about him, I suggested he mentor kids. He joined an entrepreneurs' club and started working with young people on fulfilling their own passions, and he absolutely loved it—and he ended up spending more than forty hours a week doing this kind of volunteering.

Another patient of mine was so depressed that he was talking about suicide. I told him that he needed to find something to do for himself. We discussed it at length; I became his buddy and convinced him to get psychological help. After much persuasion, he agreed to try—reluctantly—four things. He ended up joining a cooking club and fell in love with it; not just the creative process of cooking but also the community of people that came along with it. He even found a wife there (and now they both have great buddies—I'm no longer needed) and passion. My point: you will find something, and it can be the thing that lifts you up.

The biggest wall, I've found, is having preconceived notions that you shouldn't do something, for whatever reason. You shouldn't cook or go to yoga because you're a guy, you shouldn't write poetry cause you're a football player, you shouldn't enjoy competition because you're a yoga instructor, you shouldn't try swimming because you had a bad experience as an eight-year-old. Baloney. Be open to exploration, testing limits, and dipping your toe into waters that you never thought you would. Everyone has his or her passion and purpose; it just may take a while for some of us to find them.

#4 | The Magic Ingredient: Optimism

No matter what field you're in or what circles you travel in, you know there are two kinds of people: the "but" people and the "and" people. The "but" people are the ones who always find the problems in whatever is being presented. But this, but that, but but but. In contrast, the "and" people love what you say and want to build off it, creating and inspiring togetherness rather than divisiveness. I want to be with the "and" people. And so do you. (As I mentioned previously, when our kids were growing up, I banned the word *can't* in our house as the worst of all four-letter words.)

Why? Because optimistic people are healthier. So fill your glass up if it's half empty. In one study, nuns judged optimistic by their essay answers forty years prior to death lived about eight years younger (longer and with less disability) than the nuns whose essays were judged to reflect pessimism.

Likewise, the camaraderie of team play helps men lose weight. According to a study from Scotland, men who took part in a weight-loss program designed specifically for male soccer fans lost an average of twelve pounds over twelve months—and kept it off twelve months after that. Nearly 90 percent of the original participants continued the program to completion, and in a number of clubs, the men continued to meet up to exercise together after the formal program ended. They loved their teams and found that this ongoing support really helped maintain and build their motivation. These soccer fanatics were optimistic their team would win—and that optimism about the prospect of winning was contagious. It gave them confidence in other parts of their lives, and that they could get healthier. They worked hand-in-hand—optimism leading to a spirit of camaraderie and vice versa.

And remember our old pal oxytocin, the feel-good chemical that gets released when you're in a relationship with someone, romantic or not? Well, like we saw before, it seems that passion in relationships can enhance oxytocin release, optimize your resolve and motivation, and once again play a role in your Do-Over—this time, perhaps in encouraging monogamous relationships. In a 2014 study, forty heterosexual young men who had dated women for at least six months and described themselves as "madly in love" underwent a test to determine what happens in the brain when they saw images of their sweetie pies. The men were randomly assigned to inhale either oxytocin or use a nasal spray placebo (with no chemicals in it). Stationed in a brain scanner, they were then shown a series of photos: images of their romantic partners, as well as those of other women they knew or did not know. The women who were "strangers" were rated beforehand by an independent group of people to match the "objective beauty" of the female partner. So what happened?

When men who inhaled oxytocin saw the women they loved, their brains lit up like a Valentine's Day fireworks show; the desire and pleasure regions of their brains activated powerfully. By contrast, the strangers who were "equally beautiful" as their partner evoked no such response, and female friends evoked a milder version of the response to the romantic partner, suggesting that more oxytocin makes current partners more desirable. Further, the study suggests that oxytocin may actually act two ways: it makes partners more attractive at the same time that it suppresses interest in other potential mates. Notably, the men who took the placebo did not exhibit the same release of oxytocin when they saw their loved ones. This suggests that activities that increase the release of oxytocin—intimate moments, kissing, hugging, shared adventures—strengthen the relationship, making everyone optimistic.

If you're having trouble getting going, use these four steps to see if you can kick-start some of that optimism:

1 You guessed it! A daily walk of thirty to sixty minutes, aiming to get to your Do-Over goal of ten thousand steps every day, no excuses. Dispelling stress through physical activity is calming and empowering.

2 Do something special (big or small) for a friend or family member once a week. The positive feedback will start you looking forward happily to next week's interaction.

3 Practice mindful meditation for fifteen minutes a day (sitting or lying quietly, eyes closed, trying to block out all thoughts, perhaps repeating a mantra). This can help you reframe your outlook and be more present to appreciate the moment and all it has to offer.

4 Volunteer at a community center or charity; focus your attention on helping make the world better for others. The rewards you reap from giving to others are inestimable, and they can help to boost your sense of what's possible.

Now, that's not to say there shouldn't be disagreements, and that we should all live life holding hands and singing la-la-la tunes to hide our troubles. But the difference is this: the "but" people don't want solutions. They want to settle. They want to wade in their misery. The "and" people find solutions to problems. They inspire others to do their best.

They contribute to the growth of people and ideas—and, ultimately, to the health of us all.

Even if you are an avowed lifelong naysayer, the good news is you have the opportunity to discover your inner enthusiast: once you find that purpose and passion, your optimism levels rise, and your Do-Over becomes stronger and stronger and stronger. In the end, optimism is really just about cultivating happiness in your everyday, moment-to-moment life.

#5 | Passion Is Not the Same Thing as Obsession

Just a quick note here: I don't want you to think that having a passion means that you have to spend nineteen hours a day doing what you love, though you certainly can. A passion can be something you do on the weekend. A passion can be something you do a few minutes a day. A passion can be something you do once a year. The amount of time you spend is not our measuring stick; whether it drives you and what you feel and do in between those times are what count. So don't get the impression that in order to be healthy, you have to spend every waking moment collecting bottle caps. You'll do it when you can, and how you can, and in whatever quantities you can—not because you have a sense that you have to but because you'll want to. That's the driving force: the quality of your time in the moments you practice your passion, and the resulting joy that spills over into all other areas of life between those moments.

#6 | Pass It On

Purpose allows you to go above and beyond your own self-ish needs for survival. As a species, we were designed to live long enough to ensure reproduction opportunities to maximize the chance of humankind's survival. Today we live long beyond that short time frame, of course, so now it begs the question: What are we here for? I think that part of why we're here is to ensure the survival of the species in a different way—beyond a purely biological standpoint. To help others. To give wisdom to others. To inspire others. To make the world a better place for everyone, from people we care about to people we may not even know.

I'm all for so-called selfish pursuits (as in, my squash passion does nothing for other people), but I also think that the x factor in finding your lasting passion really involves how much and how deeply you can change people's lives. How can you pass along your talents, your smarts, your love to others? You can do it by starting a walking group or offering to be a buddy for someone who needs help. You can do it by volunteering, or simply sharing your knowledge (or a great healthy recipe) with someone. Giving comes in all forms, but the results are the same: selfless and soulful satisfaction. When you make that part of the equation, I believe, your Do-Over is just about as complete as it gets.

#7 | When It All Comes Together, You Inspire Others

Let me tell you the story of Tawny, who at one point was a healthy young woman. All her numbers were good, and she had a healthy weight. Things changed after going through seven years of high stressors, including the death of a brother and sister, becoming the sole caregiver of her elderly father, raising a teenage child who developed a serious illness, divorce, then becoming an empty-nester, having her family affected by the events of 9/11 . . . Any one of these would be enough to put people through high amounts of stress (remember those major life events?), but when they're all together, that's just too much for most people to reasonably handle without the consequences of some negative health outcomes. And that's what happened to Tawny. She became seriously depressed and obese.

She came (really, was sent by her family) to me for help, and I got her started—coaching her (being her buddy) on the very seven deeds I've outlined in this book, from avoiding the five food felons, to journaling food choices, to reinforcing the three values that give meaning to life (having good health, having a purpose in life, and having a life partner to share the previous two things). In six months, Tawny lost fifty pounds and gained back her good health. She was strong, beautiful, and her blood work was in great shape. But guess what happened? She didn't stop. In fact, she took the greatest step after taking her first step. When she left my office after her first appointment, she founded a walking club that meets every weekday morning at six o'clock to walk and talk for seventy-five minutes. She has been doing this for more than six years.

Because of her success and what she did with her walking club, I asked her if she wanted to join me as a coach of Enforcer eCoaching, where we coach (are buddies to) hundreds of people. This helped her achieve deed number seven: a purpose in life. (And in an uncanny turn of events, she met someone through her coaching, a potential investor in the Enforcer eCoaching company, who turned out to be the person she could share her good health and purpose with!) So she achieved not just purpose and health, but love too. Since Tawny left eCoaching, she has been asked to coach employees of small companies, many of whom didn't even speak English. She worked with one team, and over five months, the forty-seven employees lost a total of 282 pounds. She was a true buddy and coached from experience and from the heart. She passed it along to others. To this day, Tawny still says something that sticks with me: "Behaviors are contagious in a community."

This is exactly what I want you to embrace as we embark on your Do-Over. It's not about gritting your teeth and struggling. It's not about being frustrated with failures. It's not about denying yourself things to the point where you want to rebel.

It's about finding your purpose and using that to drive your choices. We get healthy because health is what gets us everything else we want in life. And once we find that out, we can't wait to share it, pass it along, inspire others, and help people find the same foundation for healthy living that we have.

I hope you've learned by now that, biologically and psychologically, a Do-Over is about forgiving past failures. It is about your future. It is a celebration of yourself. You have the power to change your body on the inside and out. So get on out there, love yourself, and live your Do-Over—and then make it your mission to help someone else live theirs.

The Plan

If you've gotten this far, or even if you've just skipped to the back of the book, you probably already know that this whole darn book is your plan. That is, each of the seven Do-Over deeds is a directive—an action to get your body to wellness, to high energy, and even to forgiveness for yesteryear's excess eggnog. All these paths lead, of course, to a new you.

This book gives you those essential strategies to do just that: get you started on your Do-Over by explaining why and how these seven deeds work. Follow those seven strategies, and you'll get your Do-Over. Simple as that.

But in my book, literally and metaphorically, a successful Do-Over is all about preparation. In fact, preparation is really the secret to instilling good habits and shielding you from temptations. We see it in nutrition (preparing your meals prevents drive-thru disasters in the heat of hunger). We see it in activity (planning a walk with a friend ensures you won't retreat to the couch). We see it in many aspects of our health and our life. So that's why this seven-day plan is really the Do-Over Preparation Plan: In just one week you build the foundation that lets you enjoy this Do-Over for your lifetime.

It's quite simple, actually. Every day for seven days, I'm

going to give you three tasks to accomplish. Do them, and you'll set yourself up to rock and roll on Day 8: to begin forming those positive habits, and to push the start button on a new approach to how you eat, how you move, and how you'll get your Do-Over. In addition, I'm going to give you some of my favorite strategies that will help you get going— and keep going. Here you'll find lots of tips and tricks that'll support you in your quest to stick with your Do-Over deeds.

Best of all, it's not that hard. Give yourself seven days to prepare, and then you're off! This is your Do-Over. Let's give it a go.

The 7-Day Do-Over Preparation Plan

Day 1

1. Order or buy a pedometer, or an app or some other device that will allow you to calculate the number of steps you take every day. You'll see my list of options on page 128. Take some time to investigate which type you prefer: something you can wear on your waistband or your bra strap or something on your phone. Ask yourself whether you need all the additional bells and whistles that may or may not come with your device. It's my experience that the simpler, the better. But this is an individual choice, and you should spend a little time researching and deciding which will be best for your technological preferences and lifestyle. As soon as you get your pedometer or device, program it to calculate your steps (even if you get it online, try to get it delivered and on you by day 4). They're usually not too complicated to set up, but it may take a few minutes to make sure it's calibrated to your step length (as well as other variables, depending on what factors you want to calculate). Keep it on for the rest of the day and record how many steps you take. Set up a log on your calendar (see step 2 of day 7) to keep track of your progress and give you the chance to take pride in your daily accomplishments. You also can use old-fashioned paper, or a tracking app, or software like Excel, or a service like Google docs if you want access to your log from multiple devices.

2. Write down (and give yourself space for answers beneath) these questions:

- What about my health or wellness has not been going how I'd like it to? (Sample answers: "I feel sluggish all day," "I'm resigned about my weight," "My blood pressure is on an upward march," "I feel good about where I am but I'm looking to get to the next level.")
- What do I want for myself with my health and wellness? In my wildest dreams, what does that look like? ("I race my grandkids to the top of the hill," "I look forward to the thrill of exercise," "I master the use of my knife," "I feel at home in my clothes again," "I win the local 5K race," "My neighbors beg to come over to eat my impossibly delicious felon-free meals.")
- What negative thought(s) or mantra(s) do I usually turn to when I think I've failed? ("I can't be

counted on," "I'm such a dummy," "I'm the worst," "It's all my fault," "It's all *their* fault," "I can't do it on my own," "Everyone's out to get me," "I'm a fat whale drowning in a sea of sadness and blubber." And so on.)

◆ What playful, positive, or relieving declaration(s) can I substitute for the less fun (and less useful) ones? ("*Wow*, I messed up—now back to it!" "I got this," "I am bigger than my neural circuitry!" "My brain's habits ain't got nothin' on *me*," "I'm a 10K-a-day-ninja," "I'm the health fairy and can't be stopped!" And so on.)

3. Make a list of five people who can be potential buddies. These can be family members, old friends, new friends, or online friends. Go with your gut on who you think would be supportive and challenging at the same time. See all my criteria in chapter 1 for what makes a good buddy. Don't contact them yet; just make a preliminary list. Don't worry about hurting feelings or choosing someone you "think you should." You need to find someone who can do this with no excess baggage involved.

Day 2

1. Buy shoes. If you don't have running or walking shoes, purchase a quality pair. A specialty running/walking store can help find a shoe that fits your gait and movement patterns to help you avoid injury. You can even get fitted for them and find discounted models online. See page 129 to see how to arrange this and what to look for.

2. Buy a knife and practice. While you are in shopping mode, buy three different kinds of vegetables that you like— you know, squash, tomatoes, and onions. (Yes, I know technically tomatoes are a fruit, but they function like a veggie in many dishes.) Whatever you like. And if you don't have a good kitchen knife, go to a kitchen store and test chef's knives (I describe a way to choose on page 185). Then buy a really high quality one. (It is one of the five things to overpay for; the other four are a pedometer, a heart rate monitor, cross training shoes, and a wedding ring.) If not too overpriced, order two on the Internet: one for you and one for your buddy. Practice chopping up all your veggies using the techniques I describe on page 186. Then go ahead and eat your work when you're done. You can make a great-tasting ratatouille.

3. Food weaknesses, part one. Write down the three felonious foods you tend to splurge on. Don't do anything with them. (Especially don't eat them!) Just write them down.

Day 3

1. Quiz yourself. Take this nutrition label quiz. Look at the label on page 312. Identify five things that indicate that this isn't the healthiest product around. (Answers on page 314.) This test will help make sure you've brushed up on nutritional guidelines so that when you're ready to shop for your everyday foods, you know how to avoid the five food felons and focus on healthy ingredients.

2. Food weaknesses, part two. Remember your list of food weaknesses? Next to each one of them, write down one thing that you can do to substitute eating them if you feel a binge coming on. It can be substituting a healthy or spicy food like roasted asparagus for French fries, or munching celery stalks with pure ground peanut butter instead of chips (the peanut butter should be a one ingredient item: peanuts only, or at most, peanuts and salt). Instead of a food substitution, you can also choose an active behavior such as stretching or walking. It can be anything. The key here is that you want to come up with contingency plans. Once that plan is in place, it's much easier to avoid temptation knowing that you have an alternative.

3. Make a shopping list and dump the pantry. Write down the healthy foods that you'll want to keep in your house— and ones that you'll need to prepare upcoming meals. (See some ideas on pages 304 and 309.) And before you go shopping (see item 1 on day 6), dump out and never replace foods from your pantry and fridge that have any of the five food felons as one of the first five ingredients. Depending on your pantry, this may be a real undertaking, so budget yourself at least an hour to scan labels and make sure you catch even the sneakiest of felons. You will have to keep some healthy foods (or even some unhealthy ones) around, otherwise you may run out of food in the next three days (before you have time allocated for food shopping—see item 1 on day 6).

Day 4

1. Get a calendar *that works for you.* Whether you've never used a calendar, you're a die-hard smartphone scheduler, or you like to use old-fashioned date books, the goal is minimally to empty out some of the frenzied to-do lists we cycle through in our brains and store them in an external support tool. Choose a calendar you will visit on a daily basis and then *actually use it* (this is critical!) to navigate your days. Now take out that calendar and make an appointment to do something that you're passionate about. That's right. Put it in your calendar. I don't care if it's a week from now, tomorrow, or in a month. But I want you to block off time for something—anything!—that *you* want to do. No questions asked from anybody else. Be selfish. Take some "me" time. If it involves other people, that's okay; take the lead to coordinate schedules and get a date on the calendar. (If you don't know what it is that you're passionate about, then do this assignment: Make a list of five things you'd like to try. Pick one—perhaps the easiest one to try out—and make a date and time to try it. Ask a friend or family member to join you, if you like.)

2. Using the criteria for choosing the ideal buddy I listed on page 81, go ahead and pick your buddy, as well as one back-up buddy. Contact your first choice, tell him or her your plans, your goals, and that you'd like to have a partnership in which you're checking in with each other (even just minimally) every day. Tell your buddy all the reasons why she is special to you—and why you think she's the one who can help you.

3. Aim to do thirty squats (see page 120 for technique) throughout the day. You can set an alarm and do three an hour every hour you are awake from eight in the morning until six in the evening. Get your body used to the fact that you'll be doing some strength training. You can even bang out a few while cooking.

Day 5

1. Solve the problem(s). Make a list of five things or issues that have nagged you for the last six months. These are not daily stresses and deadlines but things that have been hanging over your head that you have not been able to find solutions for, or that you just haven't scheduled the time to resolve. Next to each, write down possible solutions and what you would need to do to help solve them. Prioritize which ones you can handle first and then (again, this is critical) put a date in your calendar by when you will have resolved them. You do not need to solve the problems today. (I know these are not that easy.) Your goal for today is to think of strategies that will help you solve them, schedule in time to handle them, and set yourself up to successfully chip away at those nagging stresses.

2. Identify any parts of your life that feel unorganized: could be a closet, could be the de facto Post-it note calendar you've scattered throughout the house, could be bills or bank statements you've ignored for three months. Devote an hour to one area and clean it up. An organized life calms your mind and allows you to think clearly about what you need to do to get healthy. If your unorganized areas require more than an hour of attention, simply make another appointment with yourself to tackle and complete them.

3. Share some warm fuzzies. Do something nice—and unexpected—for your spouse or partner. Be creative. Do it "just because." If your relationship needs healing or work, this is a simple step in that direction. Have fun and be vulnerable: you can even ask what would be nice for them, what would make a difference to their day. If your relationship is already more fiery than a pizza oven, then, well, something else might just be part of today's to-do list. If you are single, simply do something nice for yourself or someone you care about.

Day 6

1. Go food shopping. Budget enough time to food shop for all the healthy foods and spices in the list you made on day 3. Make sure you leave the store with plenty of fruits and veggies and all the ingredients you need to prepare dinner tonight.

2. Prepare to cook your version of the ideal healthy meal for dinner tonight. While at the store, shop for it. It may take some time to experiment to find your favorites, but the purpose of trying out new recipes is for you to be able to have a meal or two or three that you can always turn to—something that's easy, quick, healthy, and tasty. Maybe it's grilled fish, steamed broccoli (drizzled with some red pepper flakes or spicy Sriracha sauce), and a few slices of avocado. Or maybe it's grilled chicken, roasted asparagus (with balsamic vinegar), and some quinoa. Mix and match how you like with a lean protein, a vegetable, healthy fat, and if you like, a 100 percent whole grain. Take some time to think about what will work for your tastes—and that of your family—so that this healthy meal (and some variations) becomes a family staple. After dinner, ask what the family thinks, and consider adjustments you can make in the future. The more of these ready-to-go meals you can prepare, the less likely you are to fall into the trap of unhealthy options.

3. Stretch for five minutes, just to give yourself a moment to relax, to breathe, to feel what it's like to allow your muscles to stretch and lengthen. This may or may not become one of your go-to stress-relieving techniques, but I really want you to feel what it's like to slow down for a moment and give your body some much-needed rejuvenation. The three I would recommend:

◆ Touch your toes. If you can't touch your toes yet, hold onto the back of your legs or calves. Bend down and hold yourself in a deep stretch. This opens up your hamstrings and back, which get tight from sitting. Do for one minute.

◆ Lie on your back and pull one knee to your chest. This opens up your hips, which are notoriously tight for so many. Switch sides. Do for one minute on each side.

◆ Stand against a wall, with one arm flat against it and behind you so that your arm is parallel to the floor. Rotate your body so you feel a stretch in your chest. This will open up your chest and help improve posture. Do for one minute on each side.

Day 7

1. Make a mantra. Remember task two from day 1? Return to your brainstorm and choose or create a favorite positive mantra; a few words that mean something to you, that show your resolve, that define what your mission is. It can be something simple like "Be bold" or "Relentless forward motion" or "Don't give up" or any few words that always seem to get you going. Use it when you need a push, some inspiration, or just a little more mojo to stay the course. It may be simple, but a few words that are *yours* can do wonders when you need them the most.

2. Up your steps. Gradually increase your steps by never doing fewer today than you did yesterday till you hit ten thousand a day, and then never go below ten thousand. Do not advance too fast: on your first day of walking keep track of the number of steps you take in a typical day. Never increase by more than five hundred steps a day, no matter how good you feel. And never advance by more than 1,500 for any day week over week (so on any day next week, your steps should never be more than 1,500 steps greater than the maximum you took any day this week), no matter how good you feel or how much you want to challenge yourself.

3. Call, text, or email your buddy with this message: "You ready? I am." When your buddy responds, start emailing or calling him or her at the end of every day with your food choices and your step number. If your buddy doesn't respond after two emails, select another buddy.

The Do-Over Deeds: Day 8 and Beyond

Community: Build a buddy system and contact your buddy every day, no excuses.

Activity: Walk ten thousand steps a day, no excuses, and do resistance exercises twice a week.

Nutrition: Arrest and ban the five food felons.

Behavior: Break the addiction, form healthy habits.

Stress: Figure out your stress solutions.

Relationships: Keep love in your life.

Passions: Explore and engage to choose your passion and purpose.

Super 7s: Great Ideas for Creating Healthy Habits

7 Easy-to-Make Do-Over Meals

◆ Egg-white omelet with grilled veggies, no cheese.

◆ Steel-cut oatmeal with blueberries and walnuts.

◆ Chopped salad and walnuts, veggies, greens, and 2 ounces of canned salmon, turkey, or chicken with balsamic vinegar.

◆ Cup of your favorite veggie soup, such as garden harvest or butternut squash carrot and ginger soup. (See the Sharecare website, at www.sharecare.com /Do-Over, for recipes—this is a website I helped start to support people in their Do-Over goals.)

◆ Veggie-stuffed 100 percent whole wheat pizza.

◆ Corn tortilla soft shell tacos with black beans, roasted beets, kale, and avocado.

◆ Mustard crusted salmon with spinach and broccoli.

7 Do-Over Stress Relievers

◆ One minute of jumping jacks (or shadow boxing: punching in the air).

◆ Ten deep breaths.

◆ Licking your lips and then blowing air on them. (It's a cooling mechanism that helps cool you down.)

◆ Writing a thank-you note or email to show your gratitude (and remind yourself of the good in the world).

◆ Five minutes of silence in a dark room, eyes closed, quietly repeating the mantra you created.

◆ Walking one thousand steps.

◆ Snacking on carrot sticks sprinkled with sea salt (like a bag of chips but without the caloric baggage).

7 Do-Over Ideas for Finding Your Passion

◆ Sign up for a continuing education course at the local community college.

◆ Start a book club (or a healthy meal club or any kind of club that meets once a month).

◆ Sign up for a goal walk or race that you can do with friends and family.

◆ Take a walk in the woods and think about what inspires you.

◆ Dance.

◆ Ask to join a friend who has found his or her passion to see if you can observe or participate. Let the inspiration hit you with this activity or give you ideas for others.

◆ Keep a journal and let the ideas flow.

7 Do-Over Ideas for Igniting More Passion in Your Relationship

◆ Communicate about areas of conflict and work to resolve them.

◆ Share household chores equally.

◆ Ask more questions, give fewer answers.

◆ Send a sexy text—but not a sext! (Unless that's your thing!)

◆ Instead of "One cooks, one cleans up," try "Cook together, clean up together."

- More shared shower time!
- Just ask what he or she would like when it comes to the bedroom department.

7 Things You Should Say to Your Do-Over Buddy

- "Great job. Keep on going."
- "Remember what you want and why you're doing this. Now let's get back on track tomorrow."
- "How's it going today?"
- "We're going to do this together!"
- "Yeah, of course I love you, but you're not helping anyone—and you're definitely not helping yourself—by ordering the grande cheese burrito."
- "Let's walk."
- "What are you having for dinner?"

7 Reasons to Do Your Do-Over
(Make Your Own List!)

- Self-respect
- Better memory
- Teach the grandkids
- Better sex
- Self-respect
- Lower health copays
- Better sex

7 Things Never to Say to Your Do-Over Buddy

◆ "You're pretty bad at this whole Do-Over thing, eh?"

◆ "Fine, Doritos boy, do whatever you want!"

◆ [*Silence*].

◆ "Whatever you want to do is fine."

◆ "Five thousand steps instead of ten thousand is okay."

◆ "You had a bad day. Four margaritas will do the trick!"

◆ "You sound sad. Can I bring over some brownies for you?"

7 Healthy Snacks, Sides, and Sweets You Can Substitute for Felons

◆ Water with slices of your favorite citrus and leaf stevia for diet soda

◆ Coffee with a little unsweetened almond milk and leaf stevia for dessert

◆ Glass of wine for dessert

◆ Celery and guac (from, at most, avocados, tomatoes, onions, cilantro, chili powder, salt, pepper, and a bit of olive oil and lime) for chips and dips

◆ Spaghetti squash for pasta

◆ 100 percent whole grains for refined carbohydrates

◆ Olive oil roasted Brussels sprouts (no bacon) for fries

8 (Sorry, Got Carried Away) Veggie-Based Entrée Ideas That Will Rock Your World

◆ Veggie bean chili: simmer equal parts chopped celery, onion, carrot, and bell peppers with pinto, kidney, and garbanzo beans, plus chili powder, oregano, and cumin.

◆ Vegan black bean or lentil burgers: buy frozen or make yourself with a little help from the Internet and some mushrooms, spinach, lentils, garlic, walnuts, and spices.

◆ Pureed fennel leek soup: just fennel, leek, potato, celery, vegetable bouillon, water, and olive oil. Serve with whole grain bread.

◆ Indian spiced kale and chickpeas: olive oil, garlic, kale, vegetable stock, coriander, cumin, masala, and chickpeas.

◆ Hummus with whole grain pita, greens, diced cucumbers, grape leaves, and brown rice.

◆ Pea soup accompanied by kale and butternut squash sautéed with onion.

◆ Veggie rice stir-fry: grab your favorite veggies—broccoli, carrots, mushrooms, bell peppers, sprouts, garlic, fresh ginger, basil—plus egg whites if you like, and stir-fry with canola oil over brown rice.

◆ Diced mango, avocado, scallion, and cilantro with lime juice and olive oil over a bed of quinoa, toasted pumpkin seeds, and arugula.

7 Physical Activities That You Should Consider Trying

- ◆ Dance classes (or any group class, like those offered at gyms)
- ◆ Swimming
- ◆ Walking stadium stairs
- ◆ Tennis (or badminton or squash!)
- ◆ Yoga
- ◆ Interval training (with a bike or treadmill—alternating between 20-second hard periods of work and 1-minute-40-second easy periods of recovery)
- ◆ Hiking

7 Do-Over Foods That Should Be Stocked in Every Kitchen

- ◆ Chicken, salmon filets, or salmon burgers ready to grill
- ◆ Cut-up vegetables ready to eat or cook
- ◆ Walnuts (for premeal snack to curb hunger during meals)
- ◆ A selection of favorite spices
- ◆ Berries (fresh or frozen)
- ◆ Quinoa or other healthy grains
- ◆ Your favorite healthy emergency food

7 Ways to Track and Quantify Your Do-Over Progress

◆ Count your steps every day.

◆ Count your servings of fruit and vegetables every day. Aim for at least seven servings.

◆ Take your blood pressure every two to three weeks.

◆ Measure your waist once a month.

◆ Weigh yourself no more than once a week, and always at the same time, first thing in the morning after you wake up. Even though you'll likely lose some weight quickly, I advise you not to get too caught up in the scale, since weights fluctuate so much. Stick to your plan, and the weight will come off.

◆ Get your body-fat percentage calculated. (Gyms often offer this service, and there are home scales that do, too.) Measure two to three times a year.

◆ Have your physician order you a complete blood test at the start and have it monitored every year. Pay close attention to lousy LDL cholesterol levels and blood glucose levels.

Mystery Label

Nutrition Facts

Serving Size 1 tbsp (15 mL)

Amount Per Serving

Calories 15   Calories From Fat   10

	% Daily Values*
Total Fat 1 g	**2%**
Saturated Fat 0 g	**0%**
Trans Fat 0 g	
Polyunsaturated Fat 0 g	
Monounsaturated Fat 0 g	
Cholesterol 0 mg	**0%**
Sodium 0 mg	**0%**
Total Carbohydrate 2 g	**1%**
Sugars 0 g	
Protein 0 g	

Not a significant source of dietary fiber, vitamin A, vitamin C, calcium, and iron.

INGREDIENTS: WATER, CORN SYRUP SOLIDS, PARTIALLY HYDROGENATED SOYBEAN AND/OR COTTONSEED OIL, AND LESS THAN 2% OF NATURAL & ARTIFICIAL FLAVORS, SODIUM CASEINATE (A MILK DERIVA-TIVE)**, MALTODEXTRIN, MONO- AND DIGLYCERIDES, DIPOTASSIUM PHOSPHATE, COLOR ADDED, CAR-RAGEENAN, DEXTROSE, SUCRA-LOSE, ACESULFAME POTASSIUM (NON-NUTRITIVE SWEETENER).

** Not a source of lactose.

Mystery Label Quiz

1. Where did the mystery label come from?
    a. Non-dairy creamer
    b. Sugar-free, fat-free frozen yogurt
    c. Five-hour energy drink
    d. Household cleaner

2. Which of the following is a marker of "wholesomeness" in this mystery food?
    a. Zero sugars!
    b. Each serving is only 15 calories.
    c. Zero sat fat!
    d. None.

3. Which of the following is *not* a felon?
    a. Dextrose
    b. Corn syrup
    c. Partially hydrogenated soybean and/or cottonseed oil
    d. Water

4. Which of these should *not* be a reason to "ban" this food?
    a. Acesulfame potassium
    b. Color added
    c. Zero protein
    d. Carrageenan

5. What could be a more healthful substitute for this food?
   a. Almond milk
   b. Full-fat sugar-sweetened homemade ice cream
   c. Coffee
   d. Organic soap

Answers

1: a. Consider the possible alternatives—and then avoid them too, unless you're cleaning the toilet bowl.

2: d. Yup. Zero sugars and zero sat fat are not indicators that a food has any nutritional value. And although there are very few calories in a single serving, note the serving size: *one tablespoon*. Think about how many servings of creamer you're likely to use at a time.

3: d. Dextrose is one of those *–oses* to avoid—it's a simple added sugar. Corn syrup is an added syrup, and partially hydrogenated oils are trans fats. *Even if the Nutrition Facts label says 0g trans fats.* That just means that one serving contains less than 0.5 grams—and when you use more than one serving at a time, that adds up quickly.

4: c. The absence of protein is not an indication that a food is harmful. Acesulfame potassium, like sucralose, is a zero-calorie sweetener. These artificial sweeteners affect your gut bacteria in a way that, over time, appears (according to one study so far) to promote insulin resistance. Added color is a chemical additive, and carrageenan is a thickening compound derived from seaweed that appears to cause inflammation and stomach problems.

5: a. As you learned from question one, this is a non-dairy creamer. Try replacing with unsweetened almond milk or soy. Sugar-sweetened homemade ice cream may have the benefit of not containing artificial sweeteners, but any way you scoop it, sugar and sat fat don't do you any good either (they kill you sweetly). Coffee would be a good replacement if this were five-hour energy—but it's not. Please don't eat organic soap.

The Do-Over Quiz: Pass It On

When you took my mini medical school courses way back at the start of the book, I promised there would be no exam. And there's not, of course, because your exam comes in the form of how you live every day—not in terms of passing or failing, but in navigating the choices you continuously confront throughout life. Life is multiple choice: In virtually everything you do, you can choose A, B, C, D, or a million more combinations. Whatever you choose will influence how you live, how you feel, and how healthy you are. The point of the book is that you will now have the knowledge and skills to choose the best answers for your body.

Now, though, I want to offer another kind of multiple-choice quiz—not to test your knowledge (okay, maybe to test your knowledge a *little*), but to give you some talking points so that you can do the ultimate good deed. That is, pass along your knowledge and inspiration to others.

So, don't think of the following thirty questions as a test. Think of them as conversation starters, cocktail-party fodder, and nuggets of fun and important information that may just be the thing that people close to you need to hear to inspire them to do their own Do-Over.

THIS IS YOUR DO-OVER

Now that you're well on your way to taking charge of your own Do-Over, you have some of the answers that those around you are seeking for their own health. Some of the questions and answers that follow may be the very place they start.

1. Why is chronic stress so damaging over time?
   a. It raises my blood sugar and adds layers of dangerous belly fat
   b. It raises my blood pressure and leads to impotence, wrinkles, and memory loss
   c. It makes me feel like I want to punch a woolly mammoth right in the nostrils
   d. All of the above

2. Why is it important to respect the bacteria in your body?
   a. They outnumber me 10 to 1—not great odds
   b. If I don't take my 10K steps a day they'll infect me
   c. If I eat foods like red meat, egg yolks, or diet soda, they produce chemicals that increase inflammation
   d. It's not important. I sneeze the buggers out.

3. Why is LDL so lousy?
   a. It patches onto arteries and limits blood flow
   b. It starts with an L, and "lousy" sounds better than "lewd and lascivious low-density lipoprotein"
   c. It causes diabetes
   d. It tastes crummier than HDL

4. Why does your body store fat?
   a. It's an anatomical winter coat for those living in cold climates

b. To keep scale manufacturers in business

c. It's saving me that extra slice of pizza for later

d. It tried storing protein, but it didn't stick

5. Fill in the blank: Fat partially comes from _____.

a. Eating fat. Duh.

b. Stress (. . . not just stress eating)

c. Eating more than three times a day

d. All of the above

6. Which of the following has the healthiest fat profile?

a. A bun-less cheeseburger hiding quietly under a bed of spinach

b. A vegetarian whole-wheat pasta dish with Alfredo sauce

c. Fresh egg or chicken salad

d. Salty olive oil-roasted asparagus

7. What's the best kind of workout you can do for your brain?

a. The Sunday crossword

b. A 30-minute jog

c. Resting it by not thinking, preferably in conjunction with a 12-hand Swedish massage

d. Mainlining 5-hour energy every hour

8. What is *not* a benefit of frequent, high-quality sex?

a. It releases oxytocin that makes you feel connected

b. If sufficiently vigorous, it can replace your 10K steps each day

    c. More and better orgasms = longer life and better health

    d. It will give you that afterglow

9. Which of the following meals will your body thank you for the most?

    a. A packaged diet bar—artificially sweetened with zero grams sugar, just five grams of saturated fat, vitamins A to Z, and more protein than a steak

    b. A steak

    c. Plain lettuce with a few tablespoons of zero-fat salad dressing and a rice cake with vegetable margarine spread for some protein

    d. A small bowl of greens, beans, and whole brown rice with walnuts, almonds, and olive oil

10. Which of the following *doesn't* stimulate oxytocin release?

    a. Sex

    b. Being with people you care about

    c. Holding a baby

    d. Oxycodone

11. Which of the following *doesn't* cause insulin resistance over time?

    a. Too much sex between lunch and dinner

    b. Too much time with chronically elevated blood sugars

    c. Too much time at the local cupcake shop

    d. Too many deadlines

12. Which of the following is true of wrinkles?
    a. They're at least partially a cardiovascular issue
    b. They can always be cured with a healthy dose of Botox
    c. They're almost always caused by the downward force of gravity
    d. You get a wrinkle for every lie you tell

13. Which of the following is *not* a food felon?
    a. Veggie 100% whole grain pizza with less than 4g sat fat from cheese
    b. Lean turkey cold cuts
    c. Roasted Brussels sprouts with pancetta
    d. A fruit smoothie made with nonfat frozen yogurt and fruit syrups

14. Buddies are to you, as Rocky is to . . .
    a. Road
    b. Mountains
    c. Bullwinkle
    d. What in the world are you talking about, doc?

15. What's a tried and true method for finding a passion?
    a. Google knows everything!
    b. Leaping into the unknown and testing something you're curious about, then testing out a second, third, or fourth pursuit.
    c. Taking a hike and reflecting for an hour about what you want to do
    d. Shrugging off your passion because you're too busy

16. Which of the following ages your arteries the most?
    a. Watching comedies on Netflix for eight hours straight, never doing any physical activity, and eating three large bags of chips each night
    b. Training for a marathon
    c. An LDL (bad) cholesterol of 240 mg/dl (normal up to 100)
    d. A pack a day of cigarettes

17. Which of the following is not like the others?
    a. Veggie lentil soup
    b. Oatmeal and berries
    c. Dark chocolate
    d. Organic grass-fed prime rib

18. Fill in the blank: Type 2 diabetes is *primarily* the result of

    _____.
    a. Type 1 evolving over time
    b. Chronic stress
    c. Too many deep-fried Oreos or similar food choices
    d. Artery clogging stimulating the release of insulin

19. Fill in the blank: Artificial zero calorie sweeteners_____

    _____.
    a. Are the Almighty's gift to mankind
    b. Settle in your kidney and cause kidney stones
    c. Promote insulin resistance and, eventually, diabetes
    d. Reduce insulin resistance, and can heal diabetes

20. Which of the following is *not* true about blood pressure?
    a. It can rise or drop depending on your level of hunger
    b. It's like pheromones—it sends out vibes that help you attract a mate
    c. It's less dependent in the long run on salt than on blood sugar
    d. It may be affected by lack of sleep

21. Which of these is *not* true about inflammation?
    a. It's always painful and only happens from injury or infection
    b. It's caused by cheeseburgers and caramel frappuccinos
    c. It decreases the likelihood you'll be having sex into your eighties
    d. More belly fat = more inflammation

22. Fill in the blank: Acute inflammation can work through

    _____.
    a. Deploying T cells to obliterate invading threats like viruses or bacteria
    b. Disorienting you and causing you to lose your bearings
    c. Switching the seat heater button in your console
    d. Giving you high lousy LDL cholesterol

23. Eating bacon several times a week is most liable to do which of the following?
    a. Cause inflammation
    b. Contribute to obesity

    c. Changes the bacteria in a vegetarian's gut within one week

    d. All of the above

24. What is the reason why most people choose to avoid gluten?

    a. It's fattening and, like other felons, causes bad belly fat

    b. They have an allergy or intolerance to it

    c. Gluten-free eating is the George Clooney of diets

    d. They're trying to firm up their glutes

25. Rank the sugar content of the following, from lowest to highest:

        I.   Three Oreos

        II. A ¼ cup of dried cranberries (Craisins)

        III. A cup of Raisin Bran

        IV. A cup of fat-free strawberry yogurt

    a. I < II < III < IV

    b. II < III < IV < I

    c. II < IV < III < I

    d. IV < III < II < I

26. Fill in the blank: Sex is important because _____.

    a. It induces insulin release, which lowers your risk for diabetes

    b. Is this an actual question?

    c. It helps you live longer and healthier, as long as it is mutually monogamous

    d. Sex is to physical activity as kale smoothies are to nutrition

27. Which of these could count toward your daily 10K steps?
    a. Sudsing up in the shower
    b. Intervals of brisk finger contractions when changing channels with the remote
    c. Meditating
    d. Kayaking

28. Which of the following could be an example of an addiction?
    a. A student who regularly skips class to play video games morning, noon, and night, who also enjoys his social life, crams before exams, and manages to scrape by with almost all A's
    b. An athlete who works out every day up to three times a day until she is injured, who then takes breaks from her training to recover fully
    c. A professional who has trouble sleeping and takes sleep medications at night (and who is now incapable of sleeping without it) and notices that he has started sleep-eating
    d. A married couple that gambles once a month to celebrate paycheck increases its visits to twice a month after the last win, then returns to the regular monthly practice the month after

29. How is addiction *different* from a bad habit?
    a. *Habit* is just a nice code word for addiction
    b. Addictions create circuitry that rewards your addictive behavior
    c. You need less and less to get the same high

    d. It causes you to eat cold turkey the day after
      Thanksgiving

30. What is the best way to celebrate your Do-Over?
    a. Pizza (made with whole-wheat crust and lots of
      veggies and no processed meats)!
    b. Call your buddy to thank her
    c. Going for a walk
    d. Finding someone you care about who you can help
      by passing along your wisdom, your motivation, your
      energy—and be a buddy to that person
    e. All of the above

Answers

1: d. The body's stress response—cultivated over evolutionary time in response to life-threatening aggressors like grumpy woolly mammoths—causes elevated blood sugar, heart rate, and blood pressure. It is a fight-or-flight response designed to enable you to escape impending danger—but if it's chronic, high sugars create their own danger: belly fat and, along with high BP, damage to your arteries. We do recommend learning how to manage chronic stress because punching your boss (today's version of the woolly mammoth) may not be as beneficial as it was when tusked beasts really were our biggest threat.

2: c. Most of your 100 trillion bacteria live in your gut where they help you to metabolize food. Red meat and egg yolks cause some of those bacteria to produce chemicals that cause major inflammation; likewise, zero-calorie sweeteners change bacteria behavior to promote insulin resistance.

3: a. Too much low-density lipoprotein (LDL) cholesterol creates patches as part of the repair process for the nicks in your artery walls. Those patches are less carefully made with higher LDL, which leads to more inflammation and larger cells and plaque in your arterial wall, less blood flow . . . which is to say, high LDLs can lead to heart attacks, stroke, impotence, and wrinkles. (Not diabetes, though!)

4: c. Even though fat can provide insulation, that's not the primary reason that we store it. When you eat more than your body needs to fuel itself—whether it's too much pizza or too many rice cakes (. . . many, many, many rice cakes)—your body shuttles those extra calories away and stores them as fat. Evolutionarily speaking, fat is a type of security blanket to make sure you have energy reserves to keep you alive in prolonged times of hunger. Evolution didn't understand that there would one day be a 7-Eleven and/or Starbucks and/or McDonald's on every other corner.

5: b. When you get down to it, eating more than you need gives you fat—but that's just one piece of the puzzle. Chronic stress elevates your circulating blood sugar, which can then be stored as belly fat. All fats—unsaturated, saturated, or trans—have the same caloric content, so eating fat alone doesn't make you fat. (However, the danger of saturated and trans fats [unlike unsaturated] is that they do not raise and may lower leptin, the hormone that turns off appetite, which makes it easier to overeat.)

6: d. Red meat, cheesy Alfredo sauce, and mayo found in egg and chicken salad are most often chock full o' saturated fats. Olive oil has some sat fats too, but unlike the others, it has a very high ratio of unsaturated fats to saturated fats—and those are the kind that you want in your diet.

7: b. Although the Sunday crossword is still a great way to increase the connectivity and strength of brain pathways, it's no match for regular aerobic exercise, which promotes BDNF (brain-derived neurotrophic growth factor), a type of Miracle-Gro that allows you to generate more powerful connections and cells in your brain's key memory area, your hippocampus.

8: b. Unfortunately, even vigorous, chandelier-swinging sex cannot fully replace those ten thousand steps—however, increased frequency of sex for men and higher quality of sex for women are linked to greater longevity and health, respectively. Another way to describe that afterglow is the oxytocin release that has you feeling happy, motivated, and connected to your partner during and after sex.

9: d. When you eat a meal you should not have to deny yourself (as in example C—lettuce and some rice cakes, plus felonious trans fatty margarine spread is not a meal). Steak is of course full of harmful carnitine and sat fats, and the diet bar is full of artificial sweeteners, sat fat, and most likely won't be that fun to eat anyway.

Greens, beans, walnuts, almonds, olive oil, and whole grain rice in small portions give your body what it needs for energy, rebuilding key tissues, reducing insulin resistance, and lengthening your stem cell telomeres. Plus, if spiced right, it just happens to taste fabulous.

10: d. Oxycodone, an opiate drug, does not stimulate oxytocin, the so-called mothering hormone. Oxytocin is released in a range of contexts where you are building a bond with someone, whether you're holding a baby, connecting with people you care about, or having sex with your partner.

11: a. As you know, stress, high blood sugars, and diets full of food felons promote insulin resistance—even if those cupcakes are sugar-free with artificial sweeteners.

12: a. Wrinkles are in fact often a cardiovascular issue—that result from blockages in certain arteries. Wrinkles on your face or arms or legs can have the same fundamental cause as a heart attack, a stroke, or a lack of blood flow to your sex organs: a blocked artery. Lack of blood flow causes loss of key supporting tissues that leads to wrinkling. While some wrinkles are caused by gravity and some are genetic, and can be treated (not cured) by Botox, they can't all be cured with an injection.

13: a. It's true—as long as the amount of pizza you're eating has fewer than 4g of sat fat, fewer than 4g of added sugars, and ideally is 100% whole grain; it is a wholesome, delicious meal. Turkey cold cuts, although they have lots of protein and less sat fats, are highly processed—and usually have harmful chemicals called nitrates. Pancetta is a fancy word for bacon (you already know the deal), and fruit smoothies that have added syrups and frozen yogurt are packed with added sugars—stick to smoothies with pure fruit and unsweetened almond or soy milk.

14: c. Yes, like Rocky and Bullwinkle, your buddy is your partner, your friend, your Batman (and your Robin) in realizing your Do-Over.

15: b. Anyone with a calendar—I'm talking the president, the ruler of the world, the parent of twelve, the CEO of a major company, folks juggling multiple jobs—can schedule a little bit of time to pursue his or her passions. Make it important to you—and you'll get more out than you put in. So B is the correct answer, unless taking a hike is your passion!

16: a. The aging your body has from sitting or lying on a couch eating chips for entertainment just is not overcome by your laughter; believe it or not, poor food choices and lack of physical activity age you more than even a pack of cigarettes every day—although that alone makes you at least ten years older.

17: d. As you may have guessed, prime rib—even the organic, grass-fed variety—is bursting with felonious carnitine (meat protein) and saturated fats. The others are felon-free: lentil soup is rich in protein and fiber, as is oatmeal, and dark chocolate has healthy polyphenols with youth-giving benefits. So the bottom line: adjust your tastes to avoid milk with fat, egg yolks, red and processed meats. This underscores the importance of adjusting your taste buds.

18: c. Type 2 diabetes can develop in a few ways, but often happens when your blood sugars are chronically elevated to a level so high that the insulin your pancreas pumps out just can't keep up—or you can also become resistant to insulin. While chronic stress is a contributor (as it also causes raised blood sugars), being overweight and a diet that gives you chronically high blood sugar are core culprits for developing the disease. By the way, if Oreos are not deep fried, the simple sugars cause the same damage, so don't reach for them either.

19: c. Artificial sweeteners may be just as damaging as other things that are known to put your body's chemical systems in a malfunctioning mode. Regular sugared beverages aren't good for you either, unless you have a wish for a slow suicide by inflammation. Try water, black coffee, or alcohol.

20: b. The fact that salt lacks big-league effects on BP (for most people without salt-sensitive hypertension) doesn't mean you can eat processed foods (in particular, processed or smoked meats) that happen to be high in salt. They are still high in other chemicals (like carnitine in red meat) that cause inflammation and considerable arterial disease. But, yes, BP has nothing to do with chemical attraction between two people, unless you meet your significant other at the BP cuff—and we haven't any reports of that.

21: a. The reason why inflammation is so tricky is that you usually can't feel it. When you are thirty-two, you may not care about having sex in your eighties, but not caring may get you into trouble well before then. (And besides which, sex is still great then too if you take care of your pipes!) You can thank me later.

22: a. In theory, inflammation is a good thing—because that's the process by which immune cells work to heal your body when threatened by injury and other invaders. The problem is, when inflammation is chronic (say when your body is trying to fight fat or cupcake overdoses or long-term stress), those systems go haywire and cause all kinds of bad effects in your body.

23: d. Red meat, meaning meat from four-legged animals, does all of those bad things. That may be why a friend in urology has dubbed the bacon-topped burger the "erectile dysfunctionator."

24: b. Gluten is a protein found in wheat, rye, and barley flours (as well as triticale and spelt). Some people suffer from an autoimmune disease (celiac) that is exacerbated by gluten, while others have more or less severe intolerances. Gluten may have some inflammatory properties, but unless you truly have celiac disease, or are allergic to it (a few tests will help let you know), you don't need to completely avoid gluten.

25: a. Yup, it's true: three Oreos contain less sugar (14g) than any other option here—and that doesn't mean you should eat them! Beware of sugar-dense foods like dried fruit (Craisins have 18g sugar per quarter cup), cereals (Post Raisin Bran has 20g per cup), and flavored yogurts (Chobani's strawberry Greek yogurt and comparable brands have about 23g sugar per cup). To put this in context, a dry ½ cup of plain whole rolled oats for oatmeal has 1g of sugar, versus a tall Starbucks Frappuccino, which has 32g. Try kissing your significant other instead of choosing any of these—much sweeter anyway.

26: c. Multiple studies from Great Britain and the US National Social Life, Health, and Aging Project show strong correlations between mutually monogamous sex and longevity . . . from better quality orgasms for women and more orgasm frequency for men.

27: d. Any form of active physical movement that's a bit more strenuous than using the remote control or taking a bath can count toward your 10K a day. Kayaking (as long as you're actually paddling!) is one great activity of many.

28: c. Remember, an addiction is not a habit. And as long as an unhealthy habit can be controlled or curtailed, it's not an addiction. So, for something to really be considered an addiction, there have to be long-term adverse consequences, as well as an increased tolerance to the substance or behavior, which is the case of the professional who starts sleep-eating.

29: b. You need more and more of the addictive substance or behavior to get the same effect—and you continue to do it despite more adverse consequences. The latter creates circuitry in your brain, so that it becomes easier to choose the addiction, just as it is easier to play "Chopsticks" the more you do it. To break the addiction you need to prune the circuit, which takes more time than eating a turkey, even a one-day-old cold turkey. So, cold turkey doesn't work as well as building up an alternative behavior in place of the addictive habit over many months.

30: e. But you already knew that.

Acknowledgments

This work is the product of the education I've received since 1987 coaching over 10,000 people to help them get their Do-Overs. Almost every individual I've worked with has taught me something unique about health and about life. Undoubtedly, the most important lesson is that the key to getting a Do-Over is recruiting the right buddy.

I am first and always indebted to these individuals for teaching me so much and for motivating me with their insights as they underwent their Do-Overs—and changed their lives in the process. Almost all of the people cited in the book had their names altered in the text to protect their privacy. But the names of the lead coaches with whom I have worked recently are real. Tawny Ratner and Amy Gannon have tirelessly impressed upon me the importance of selecting just the right coach—just the right buddy—for each person. Our chief CIO for the program, Percy Bhathena, has kept me focused on that—that is why I need to acknowledge these three up-front.

I am fortunate to work with such a talented and creative group as my partner in much of RealAge and coaching, Dr. Keith Roach, and the family that taught me about writing and much more, Lisa and Mehmet Oz. Thank you for your partnership.

Learning and updating the science behind Do-Overs demanded a true team effort—one that blended the talents, creativity, thoughts, and wisdom of many. It all began long ago when we realized that complications after surgery increase dramatically as you age. It became my mission to discover ways to essentially reverse the aging process. I am indebted to our wonderful collaborators at RealAge.com, now Sharecare.com, including medical lead Axel Goetz, CEO Charlie Silver, and its late cofounder, Marty Rom, who fostered this effort from the beginning. The RealAge metric is now updated and made even more relevant with bold leadership and a buddy matchup by Jeff Arnold, pushed by Dawn Whaley, Russ Johannesson, and Dermot Waters at Sharecare.com.

The Anesthesiology, Critical Care, and Pain Management Institute that I led at the Cleveland Clinic wanted to do more than draw blood and test it before surgery—we wanted to make our patients ten years younger in the two weeks surrounding their procedures so that they wouldn't need our intensive-care services afterward. That is what we did and do daily to many as a result of this work. The clinic CEO, Toby Cosgrove, took the position that the Cleveland Clinic cannot continue to do just illness care and consider itself a great institution or enable its caregivers to thrive. Dr. Cosgrove has said that while the clinic has been and will continue to be known as one of the best, if not the best, in illness care, wellness is part and parcel of what the clinic does and must do for every employee and every person we touch.

ACKNOWLEDGMENTS

Many others contributed more than they know, including Martin Harris, Caldwell Esselstyn Jr., John LaPuma, Mark Rudberg, Mladen Golubic, Rich Lang, Raul Seballos, Steve Feinleib, Roxanne Sukol, Melissa Young, Lyla Blake, Dan Neides, Adam Bernstein, Andy Bang, chef Jim Perko, Kristin Kirkpatrick, Jennifer Hunter, Judi Barr, Jane Ehrman, and many other nutritionists, stress therapists, and exercise physiologists. In a book of this scope based in science, no one human (at least not this one) commands all the needed knowledge, so I sought advice from many world experts who selflessly shared their insights in the true academic tradition, including Dean Ornish, Mark Hyman, Daniel Amen, and Jean Chatzky (who slogged through reading the manuscript still in "word form" to write blurbs); Regina Chandler, Joe Hahn, Brian Donley, Mike Modic, Kelly Hancock, Jim Young, David Longworth, Tony Miniaci, Linda McHugh, Jim Merlino, Abby Abelson, Val Weaver, Kalia Doner, Sari Harrar, Laurie Herr, Len Calabrese, Michael Gershon, Tracy Hafen, Jon Lapook, Arthur Perry, Paul Rosenberg, Zeyd Ebraham, Lilian Gonsalves, Roz Wattell, Jennifer Ashton, Linda Bradley, Glen Copeland, Nancy Foldvary, Bryon Hoogwerf, Gordon Hughes, Susan Joy, Cynthia Kubu, Allison Vidimos, Michael Breus, Bob Uttl, Bruce N. Ames, Jim Zacny; and those who inspire, such as Reverend Otis Moss, Muriel Alexandrowski, Mary Pipino, Bud Isaacson, Bridget Duffy, and Albert and Audrey Ratner. I know I am leaving some out. And most importantly, I am fortunate to work with many nurses and caregivers who have broken traditional molds and are making the Cleveland Clinic the best place to work and the best place to receive care—and who, by honoring wellness as a culture and value, are living the future of healthcare.

Our family was fully engaged: Jennifer, Jeff, Sydney, and Nancy were critical readers; so was my sister, Marsha Lowry. They were joined at times by the "extended family" of the Katzes, Unobskeys, and Campodonicos. I also need to thank Sukie Miller, Craig Wynett, Linda Defrancisco, Carl Peck, Eileen Sheil, and John Maudlin for helping start and encourage this type of work, and many on the RealAge team who validated and verified the content and contributed their expertise to the book.

I thank agent Candice Fuhrman's honest commentary and tough advice, which allowed this manuscript to mature into the book America deserves. Her editor, Karie Jacobson, was brutally frank, but that made the book much better. I thank Olivia R. Delia who worked tirelessly on multiple revisions of this book, as well as on the script to spread the word, which will be used for the PBS special of the same name. Without Olivia, *This Is Your Do-Over* would be a far inferior product

I also want to thank insightful editor Shannon Welch at Scribner (Simon & Schuster) who so enthusiastically supported this material and whose team dedicated itself to bringing these ideas to the world. I want to thank Diane Reverand—she started this process by telling me not to worry about offending medical colleagues. And I couldn't have done this at all without the scheduling prowess of Beth Grubb, who also made the plan much more time efficient.

Ted Spiker is one of the most unique people I have ever had the honor of working with. Ted deserves a doctorate from our mini medical school, plus a hall of fame award in journalism. He is a true master of his craft, taking whatever I write or say and putting it in fun-to-read prose that describes difficult concepts with enviable lucidity.

Only my wife, Nancy, deserves more praise for her continuing patience and inspiration—marrying her was the best thing I did, and it made me a much better physician.

I hope you, the reader, benefit from her encouragement and belief in the central mission of this book—to help you understand that if you want one, you can have and deserve a Do-Over.

From Ted Spiker

My deepest thanks to Dr. Michael Roizen for entrusting me with his message, his work, and his mission to improve the health of the world. Working with Mike is a true joy, because not only does his brain have the capacity of a zillion-gig hard drive, but also because he cares about every single person he comes in contact with. While he'll likely never forgive me for occasionally straying into the land of meatballs and mashed potatoes (not usually at the same time), I will always value all I have learned from him about health, wellness, and spreading the word of healthy living. Getting to work with Mike now, as well as with him during our run of *YOU: The Owner's Manual* books with Dr. Mehmet Oz, has been one of my career highlights.

Also, I must thank all of my colleagues and students at the University of Florida, as well as my friends and fam-

ACKNOWLEDGMENTS

ily for their continued support of my endeavors. So many people have played a role in helping in my writing and teaching career.

Most of all, my deepest gratitude goes to my wife, Liz, and my boys, Alex and Thad, for their love, patience, enthusiasm, and support. My wedding day and the birth of my boys were the two greatest days of my life—not just because of what happened on those days, but for every day after.

Index

INDEX

INDEX

INDEX

INDEX

INDEX

INDEX

INDEX

INDEX

INDEX